EVIDENCE-BASED TREATMENT PLANNING FOR DISRUPTIVE CHILD AND ADOLESCENT BEHAVIOR

EVIDENCE–BASED TREATMENT PLANNING FOR DISRUPTIVE CHILD AND ADOLESCENT BEHAVIOR

DVD COMPANION WORKBOOK

ARTHUR E. JONGSMA, JR.
AND
TIMOTHY J. BRUCE

WILEY

John Wiley & Sons, Inc.

ISBN 978-0-470-56858-3

Printed in the United States of America

10 9 8 7 6 5 4 3 2 1

Contents

Introduction   vii

Chapter 1   What Are the Disruptive Behavior Disorders?   1

Chapter 2   What Are the Six Steps in Building a
Psychotherapy Treatment Plan?   5

Chapter 3   What Is the Brief History of the Empirically
Supported Treatments Movement?   7

Chapter 4   What Are the Identified Empirically Supported
Treatments for the Disruptive Behavior Disorders?   12

Chapter 5   How Do You Integrate Empirically Supported
Treatments Into Treatment Planning?   31

Chapter 6   What Are Common Considerations for
Relapse Prevention?   50

Closing Remarks and Resources   53

Appendix A   A Sample Evidence-Based Treatment
Plan for Disruptive Behavior   55

Appendix B   Chapter Review Test Questions and
Answers Explained   59

Introduction

This *Workbook* is a companion to the Evidence-Based Treatment Planning for Disruptive Child and Adolescent Behavior DVD, which is focused on informing mental health therapists, addiction counselors, and students in these fields about evidence-based psychological treatment planning.

Organization

In this *Workbook* you will find in each chapter:

- ➤ Summary highlights of content shown in the DVD
- ➤ Chapter review discussion questions
- ➤ Chapter review test questions
- ➤ Chapter references

In appropriate chapters, the references are divided into those for *empirical support*, those for *clinical resources*, and those for *bibliotherapy resources*. Empirical support references are selected studies or reviews of the empirical work supporting the efficacy of the treatments discussed in the chapter. The clinical resources are books, manuals, or other resources for clinicians that describe the application, or "how to," of the treatments discussed. The bibliotherapy resources are selected publications and Web sites relevant to the DVD content that may be helpful to clinicians, clients, or laypersons.

Examples of client homework are included at www.wiley.com/go/disruptivewb. They are designed to enhance understanding of therapeutic interventions, in addition to being potentially useful clinically.

Appendix A contains an example of an evidence-based treatment plan for disruptive child/adolescent behavior. In Appendix B, correct and incorrect answers to all chapter review test questions are explained.

Chapter Points

This DVD is electronically marked with chapter points that delineate the beginning of discussion sections throughout the program. You may skip to any one of these chapter points on the DVD by clicking on the forward arrow. The chapter points for this program are as follows:

> ➤ Defining Disruptive Behavior
> ➤ Six Steps to Building a Treatment Plan
> ➤ Brief History of the EST Movement
> ➤ ESTs for Disruptive Behavior
> ➤ Integrating ESTs for Disruptive Behavior into Treatment Planning
> ➤ Common Considerations in Relapse Prevention
> ➤ An Evidence-Based Treatment Plan for Disruptive Behavior

Series Rationale

Evidence-based practice (EBP) is steadily becoming the standard of mental health care, as it has of medical health care. Borrowing from the Institute of Medicine's definition (Institute of Medicine, 2001), the American Psychological Association (APA) has defined EBP as "the integration of the best available research with clinical expertise in the context of patient characteristics, culture, and preferences" (American Psychological Association Presidential Task Force on Evidence-Based Practice [APA], 2006).

Professional organizations such as the American Psychological Association, the National Association of Social Workers, and the American Psychiatric Association, as well as consumer organizations such as the National Alliance for the Mentally Ill (NAMI), are endorsing EBP. At the federal level, a major joint initiative of the National Institute of Mental Health and the Department of Health and Human Services Substance Abuse and Mental Health Services Administration (SAMHSA) focuses on promoting, implementing, and evaluating evidence-based mental health programs and practices within state mental health systems (APA, 2006). In some practice settings, EBP is even becoming mandated. It is clear that the call for evidence-based practice is being increasingly sounded.

Unfortunately, many mental health care providers cannot or do not stay abreast of results from clinical research and how these results can inform their practices. Although it has rightfully been argued that the relevance of some research to the clinician's needs is weak, there are products of clinical research whose efficacy has been well-established and whose effectiveness in the community setting has received support. Clinicians and clinicians-in-training interested in empirically informing their treatments could benefit from educational programs that make this goal more easily attainable.

This series of DVDs and companion workbooks is designed to introduce clinicians and students to the process of empirically informing their psychotherapy treatment plans. The series begins with an introduction to the efforts to identify research-supported treatments and how the products of these efforts can be used to inform treatment planning. The other programs in the series focus on empirically informed treatment planning for each of several commonly seen clinical problems. In each problem-focused DVD, issues involved in defining or diagnosing the presenting problem are reviewed. Research-supported treatments for the problem are described, as well as the process used to identify them. Viewers are then systematically guided through the process of creating a treatment plan, and shown how the plan can be informed by goals, objectives, and interventions consistent with those of the identified research-supported treatments. Example vignettes of selected interventions are also provided.

This series is intended to be educational and informative in nature and not meant to be a substitute for clinical training in the specific interventions discussed and demonstrated. References to empirical support of the treatments described, clinical resource material, and training opportunities are provided.

Presenters

Dr. Art Jongsma is the Series Editor and co-author of the Practice*Planners*® Series published by John Wiley & Sons. He has authored or co-authored more than

Exhibit I.1   Dr. Tim Bruce and Dr. Art Jongsma

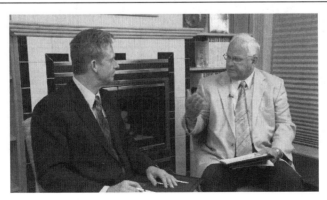

40 books in this series. Among the books included in this series are the highly regarded *The Complete Adult Psychotherapy Treatment Planner, The Adolescent Treatment Planner, The Child Psychotherapy Treatment Planner,* and *The Addiction Treatment Planner.* All of these books, along with *The Severe and Persistent Mental Illness Treatment Planner, The Family Therapy Treatment Planner, The Couples Psychotherapy Treatment Planner, The Older Adult Psychotherapy Treatment Planner,* and *The Veterans and Active Duty Military Psychotherapy Treatment Planner,* are informed with objectives and interventions that are supported by research evidence.

Dr. Jongsma also created the clinical record management software tool Thera*Scribe*®, which uses point-and-click technology to easily develop, store, and print treatment plans, progress notes, and homework assignments. He has conducted treatment planning and software training workshops for mental health professionals around the world.

Dr. Jongsma's clinical career began as a psychologist in a large private psychiatric hospital. After working in the hospital for about 10 years, he then transitioned to outpatient work in his own private practice clinic, Psychological Consultants, in Grand Rapids, Michigan for 25 years. He has been writing best-selling books and software for mental health professionals since 1995.

Dr. Timothy Bruce is a Professor and Associate Chair of the Department of Psychiatry and Behavioral Medicine at the University of Illinois College of Medicine in Peoria, Illinois, where he also directs medical student education. He is a licensed clinical psychologist who completed his graduate training at SUNY-Albany, under the mentorship of Dr. David Barlow, and his residency training at Wilford Hall Medical Center, under the direction of Dr. Robert Klepac. In addition to maintaining an active clinical practice at the university, Dr. Bruce has authored numerous publications, including books, professional journal articles, book chapters, and professional educational materials, many on the topic of evidence-based practice. Most recently, he has served as the developmental editor empirically informing Dr. Jongsma's best-selling Practice*Planners*® Series.

Dr. Bruce is also Executive Director of the Center for Evidence-Based Mental Health Practices, a state- and federally funded initiative to disseminate evidence-based psychological and pharmacological practices across Illinois. Highly recognized as an educator, Dr. Bruce has received nearly two dozen awards for his teaching of students and professionals during his career.

References

American Psychological Association Presidential Task Force on Evidence-Based Practice (2006). Evidence-based practice in psychology. *American Psychologist, 61,* 271–285.

Berghuis, D., Jongsma, A., & Bruce, T. (2006). *The severe and persistent mental illness treatment planner* (2nd ed.). Hoboken, NJ: Wiley.

Dattilio, F., Jongsma, A., & Davis, S. (2009). *The family therapy treatment planner* (2nd ed.). Hoboken, NJ: Wiley.

Institute of Medicine. (2001). *Crossing the quality chasm: A new health system for the 21st century.* Washington, DC: National Academy Press.

Jongsma, A. Peterson, M., & Bruce, T. (2006). *The complete adult psychotherapy treatment planner* (4th ed.). Hoboken, NJ: Wiley.

Jongsma, A., Peterson, M., McInnis, W. & Bruce, T. (2006a). *The adolescent psychotherapy treatment planner* (4th ed.). Hoboken, NJ: Wiley.

Jongsma, A., Peterson, M., McInnis, W., & Bruce, T. (2006b). *The child psychotherapy treatment planner* (4th ed.). Hoboken, NJ: Wiley.

Moore, B., & Jongsma, A. (2009). *The veterans and active duty military psychotherapy treatment planner.* Hoboken, NJ: Wiley.

Perkinson, R., Jongsma, A., & Bruce, T. (2009). *The addiction treatment planner* (4th ed.). Hoboken, NJ: Wiley.

What Are the Disruptive Behavior Disorders?

Defining Disruptive Behavior

Diagnostically speaking, disruptive behavior disorders refer to oppositional defiant disorder (ODD), conduct disorder (CD), and disruptive behavior disorder (NOS). Although attention deficit with hyperactivity disorder (ADHD) is a disorder characterized by disruptive behavior, it has been distinguished from the other disruptive behavior disorders and, for the most part, has its own outcome literature as well as evidence-based practice guidelines. Consistent with this distinction in the literature, we are going to focus on disruptive behavior of the oppositional and conduct type.

Having said this, please note that many of the participants in the treatment studies supporting empirically supported treatments (ESTs) for ODD and CD have multiple comorbidities, including and not limited to ADHD. Although not desirable from a diagnostic-clarity perspective, one benefit of this complexity is that it increases confidence that the research participants who have responded to ESTs for disruptive behavior are highly representative of those seen in everyday practice.

Let's look at the diagnostic criteria for the two primary disruptive behavior disorders that will be the focus of this program: ODD and CD.

Oppositional Defiant Disorder

Oppositional defiant disorder refers to a pattern of negativistic, hostile, and defiant behavior in persons less than 18 years old that lasts at least six months, during which four (or more) of the following behaviors are evident:

> Often loses temper
> Often argues with adults
> Often actively defies or refuses to comply with adults' requests or rules
> Often deliberately annoys people

> Often blames others for his or her mistakes or misbehavior
> Is often touchy or easily annoyed by others
> Is often angry and resentful
> Is often spiteful or vindictive.

These behaviors occur more frequently than is typically observed in individuals of comparable age and developmental level.

To meet criteria for ODD, the disruptive behavior should cause clinically significant impairment in social, academic, or occupational functioning.

It is also important to rule out that the disruptive behavior is not occurring exclusively during the course of a psychotic or mood disorder, and that it doesn't meet the criteria for CD.

Conduct Disorder

Conduct disorder is a more serious pattern of repetitive and persistently defiant behaviors in which the basic rights of others or major age-appropriate societal norms or rules are violated. It is characterized by the presence of three (or more) of the following criteria in the past 12 months, with at least one criterion present in the past 6 months in an individual under the age of 18:

Aggression to people and animals

> Often bullies, threatens, or intimidates others
> Often initiates physical fights
> Has used a weapon that can cause serious physical harm to others (e.g., a bat, brick, broken bottle, knife, gun)
> Has been physically cruel to people
> Has been physically cruel to animals
> Has stolen while confronting a victim (e.g., mugging, purse snatching, extortion, armed robbery)
> Has forced someone into sexual activity

Destruction of property

> Has deliberately engaged in fire setting with the intention of causing serious damage
> Has deliberately destroyed others' property (other than by fire setting)

Deceitfulness or theft

> Has broken into someone else's house, building, or car
> Often lies to obtain goods or favors or to avoid obligations (i.e., "cons" others)

➤ Has stolen items of nontrivial value without confronting a victim (e.g., shoplifting, but without breaking and entering; forgery)

Serious violations of rules

➤ Often stays out at night despite parental prohibitions, beginning before age 13 years
➤ Has run away from home overnight at least twice while living in parental or parental surrogate home (or once without returning for a lengthy period)
➤ Is often truant from school, beginning before age 13 years

The disruptive behavior causes clinically significant impairment in social, academic, or occupational functioning.

The diagnostician also specifies the onset of the disorder as follows:

➤ *Childhood-onset type*: This means that at least one criterion characteristic of conduct disorder was evident prior to age 10 years.
➤ *Adolescent-onset type*: This means there was an absence of any criteria prior to age 10 years.

Severity of the disorder is also specified as follows:

➤ *Mild*: Few if any conduct problems in excess of those required to make the diagnosis; conduct problems cause only minor harm to others
➤ *Moderate*: The number of conduct problems and their effect on others intermediates between mild and severe
➤ *Severe*: Many conduct problems, in excess of those required to make the diagnosis, or conduct problems cause considerable harm to others

ODD typically begins before the age of 8 and almost always by early adolescence.

CD usually occurs before late childhood or early adolescence, but can begin in those as young as 5 or 6 years old.

ODD has been found to be comorbid with attention deficit hyperactive disorder in 54 to 67% of children diagnosed with ADHD. CD is a more serious behavior disorder and a known precursor to antisocial personality disorder.

Chapter Review

1. What are the disruptive behavior disorders?
2. What is oppositional defiant disorder (ODD)?
3. What is conduct disorder (CD)?

Chapter Review Test Questions

1. To meet diagnostic criteria such as those in the DSM, what is the minimum length of time that the behavioral characteristics of oppositional defiant disorder (ODD) should be seen in the child?
   A. One month
   B. One year
   C. Six months
   D. Three months

2. Which of the following is a potentially severe disruptive child/adolescent behavior disorder in which there is often serious violation of the rights of others?
   A. Attention deficit disorder (ADD)
   B. Conduct disorder (CD)
   C. Oppositional defiant disorder (ODD)
   D. Separation anxiety disorder (SAD)

Chapter Reference

American Psychiatric Association. (2000). *Diagnostic and statistical manual of mental disorders* (4th ed., text revised). Washington, DC: American Psychiatric Association.

2

What Are the Six Steps in Building a Psychotherapy Treatment Plan?

Step 1: Identify primary and secondary problems
> ➤ Use evidence-based psychosocial assessment procedures to determine the most significant problem or problems related to current distress, disability, or both.

Step 2: Describe the problem's manifestations (symptom pattern)
> ➤ Note how the problem(s) is evident in your particular client. These features may correspond to the diagnostic criteria for the problem.

Step 3: Make a diagnosis based on DSM/ICD criteria
> ➤ Based on an evaluation of the client's complete clinical presentation, determine the appropriate diagnosis using the process and criteria described in the DSM or the ICD.

Step 4: Specify long-term goals
> ➤ These goal statements need not be crafted in measurable terms, but are broader and indicate a desired general positive outcome of treatment.

Step 5: Create short-term objectives
> ➤ Objectives for the client to achieve should be stated in measurable or observable terms so accountability is enhanced.

Step 6: Select therapeutic interventions
> ➤ Interventions are the actions of the clinician within the therapeutic alliance designed to help the client accomplish the treatment objectives. There should be at least one intervention planned for each client objective.

Key Point

One important aspect of effective treatment planning is that each plan should be tailored to the individual client's particular problems and needs. Treatment plans should not be boilerplate, even if clients have similar problems. Consistent with the definition of an evidence-based practice, the individual's strengths and weaknesses, unique stressors, cultural and social network, family circumstances, and symptom patterns must be considered in developing a treatment strategy. Clinicians should rely on their own good clinical judgment and plan a treatment that is appropriate for the distinctive individual with whom they are working.

Chapter Review

1. What are the six steps involved in developing a psychotherapy treatment plan?

Chapter Review Test Questions

1. Although all are disruptive, children with ODD may be disruptive in different ways. For example, some may argue and defy adults predominately, while others may deliberately annoy and blame peers. In which step of treatment planning would you record the particular expressions of ODD for your client?
   A. Creating short-term objectives
   B. Describing the problem's manifestations
   C. Identifying the primary problem
   D. Selecting treatment interventions

2. The statement, "Learn Parent Management techniques to identify and reinforce the child's desirable behavior," is an example of which of the following steps in a treatment plan?
   A. A primary problem
   B. A short-term objective
   C. A symptom manifestation
   D. A treatment intervention

Chapter References

American Psychological Association Presidential Task Force on Evidence-Based Practice. (2006). Evidence-based practice in psychology. *American Psychologist, 61*, 271–185.

Jongsma, A. (2005). Psychotherapy treatment plan writing. In G. P. Koocher, J. C. Norcross, and S. S. Hill (Eds.), *Psychologists' desk reference* (2nd ed., pp. 232–236). New York, NY: Oxford University Press.

Jongsma, A., Peterson, M., & Bruce, T. (2006). *The complete adult psychotherapy treatment planner* (4th ed.). Hoboken, NJ: Wiley.

Jongsma, A., Peterson, M., McInnis, W., & Bruce, T. (2006a). *The adolescent psychotherapy treatment planner* (4th ed.). Hoboken, NJ: Wiley.

Jongsma, A., Peterson, M., McInnis, W., & Bruce, T. (2006b). *The child psychotherapy treatment planner* (4th ed.). Hoboken, NJ: Wiley.

3

What Is the Brief History of the Empirically Supported Treatments Movement?

In the United States, the effort to identify empirically supported treatments (ESTs) began with an initiative of the American Psychological Association's Division 12, The Society of Clinical Psychology.

In 1993, APA's Division 12 President David Barlow initiated a task group, chaired by Diane Chambless. The group was charged to review the psychotherapy outcome literature to identify psychological treatments whose efficacy had been demonstrated through clinical research. This group was originally called the Task Force on the Promotion and Dissemination of Psychological Procedures and was later reorganized under the Task Force on Psychological Interventions.

Process Used to Identify ESTs

Reviewers established two primary sets of criteria for judging the evidence base supporting any particular therapy. One was labeled *well-established*, the other *probably efficacious* (Figure 3.1).

Figure 3.1

Specific Criteria for Well-Established and Probably Efficacious Treatments

Criteria for a Well-Established Treatment

For a psychological treatment to be considered *well-established*, the evidence base supporting it had to be characterized by the following:

I. At least two, good between group design experiments demonstrating efficacy in one or more of the following ways:

  A. Superior (statistically significantly so) to pill or psychological placebo or to another treatment

  B. Equivalent to an already established treatment in experiments with adequate sample sizes

(continued)

OR

II. A large series of single case design experiments (n > 9) demonstrating efficacy. These experiments must have:

   A. Used good experimental designs

   B. Compared the intervention to another treatment, as in IA

Further Criteria for Both I and II

III. Experiments must be conducted with treatment manuals.

IV. Characteristics of the client samples must be clearly specified.

 V. Effects must have been demonstrated by at least two different investigators or investigating teams.

Criteria for a Probably Efficacious Treatment

For a psychological treatment to be considered *probably efficacious*, the evidence base supporting it had to meet the following criteria:

  I. Two experiments showing the treatment is superior (statistically significantly so) to a waiting-list control group.

OR

 II. One or more experiments meeting the well-established treatment criteria IA or IB, III, and IV, but not V.

OR

III. A small series of single case design experiments (n > 3) otherwise meeting Well-Established Treatment

---

Adapted from "Update on Empirically Validated Therapies, II," by D. L. Chambless, M. J. Baker, D. H. Baucom, L. E. Beutler, K. S. Calhoun, P. Crits-Christoph, . . . S. R. Woody, 1998, *The Clinical Psychologist, 51*(1), 3–16.

Key Point

Division 12's criteria for a well-established treatment are similar to the standards used by the United States Food and Drug Administration (FDA) to evaluate the safety and efficacy of proposed medications. The FDA requires demonstration that a proposed medication is significantly superior to a nonspecific control treatment (a pill placebo) in at least two randomized controlled trials conducted by independent research groups. Division 12's criteria for a well-established treatment requires the equivalent of this standard as well as other features relevant to judging a psychological treatment's efficacy (e.g., a clear description of the treatment and study participants). By extension, if the FDA were to evaluate psychotherapies using the criteria they use for medication, it would allow sale of those judged to be well-established.

Products of Empirically Supported Treatment Reviews

The products of these reviews can be found in the Division 12 groups' final two reports.

- ➤ In the first report, 47 ESTs are identified (Chambless, et al., 1996).
- ➤ In the final report, the list had grown to 71 ESTs (Chambless, et al., 1998).
- ➤ In 1999, The Society of Clinical Psychology, Division 12, took full ownership of maintaining the growing list. The current list and information center can be found on its Web site at: www.psychologicaltreatments.org.

Around this same time, other groups emerged, using the same or similar criteria, to review literatures related to other populations, problems, and interventions. Examples include the following:

- ➤ Children (Lonigan & Elbert, 1998)
- ➤ Pediatric Psychology (Spirito, 1999)
- ➤ Older Adults (Gatz, 1998)
- ➤ Adult, Child, Marital, Family Therapy (Kendall & Chambless, 1998).
- ➤ Psychopharmacology and Psychological Treatments (Nathan & Gorman, 1998; 2002; 2007)

For those interested in comparing and contrasting the criteria used by various review groups, see Chambless and Ollendick (2001).

TherapyAdvisor

Descriptions of the treatments identified through many of these early reviews, as well as references to the empirical work supporting them, clinical resources, and training opportunities, can be found at www.therapyadvisor.com. This resource was developed by Personal Improvement Computer Systems (PICS) with funding from the National Institute of Mental Health and in consultation with members of the original Division 12 task groups. Information found on TherapyAdvisor is provided by the primary author/researcher(s) of the given EST.

Selected Organizational Reviewers of Evidence-Based Psychological Treatments and Practices

- ➤ The United Kingdom is on the forefront of the effort to identify evidence-based treatments and develop guidelines for practice. The latest products of their work can be found on the Web site for the National Institute for Health and Clinical Excellence (NICE): www.nice.org.uk.

➤ The Substance Abuse and Mental Health Service Administration, or SAMHSA, has an initiative to evaluate, identify, and provide information on various mental health practices. Their work, entitled "The National Registry of Evidence-based Programs and Practices or NREPP," can be found online at www.nrepp.samhsa.gov.

➤ The Agency for Health Care Policy and Research, now called the Agency for Healthcare Research and Quality (AHRQ) has established guidelines and criteria for identifying evidence-based practices and provides links to evidence-based clinical practice guidelines for various medical and mental health problems at www.ahrq.gov/clinic/epcix.htm.

Chapter Review

1. How did Division 12 of the APA identify ESTs?
2. What are the primary differences between *well-established* and *probably efficacious* criteria used to identify ESTs?
3. Where can information about ESTs and evidence-based practices be found?

Chapter Review Test Questions

1. Which statement best describes the process used to identify ESTs?

   A. Consumers of mental health services nominated therapies.
   B. Experts came to a consensus based on their experiences with the treatments.
   C. Researchers submitted their works.
   D. Task groups reviewed the literature using clearly defined selection criteria for ESTs.

2. Based on the differences in their criteria, in which of the following ways are well-established treatments different than those classified as probably efficacious?

   A. Only probably efficacious treatments allowed the use of a single case design experiment.
   B. Only well-established treatments allowed studies comparing the treatment to a psychological placebo.
   C. Only well-established treatments required demonstration by at least two different, independent investigators or investigating teams.
   D. Only well-established treatments allowed studies comparing the treatment to a pill placebo.

Chapter References

Chambless, D. L., & Ollendick, T. H. (2001). Empirically supported psychological interventions: Controversies and evidence. *Annual Review of Psychology, 52,* 685–716.

Chambless, D. L., Sanderson, W. C., Shoham, V., Bennett Johnson, S., Pope, K. S., Crits-Christoph, P., . . . McCurry, S. (1996). An update on empirically validated therapies. *The Clinical Psychologist, 49,* 5–18.

Chambless, D. L., Baker, M. J., Baucom, D. H., Beutler, L. E., Calhoun, K. S., Crits-Christoph, P., . . . Woody, S. R. (1998). Update on empirically validated therapies, II. *The Clinical Psychologist, 51,* 3–16.

Gatz, M., Fiske, A., Fox, L. S., Kaskie, B., Kasl-Godley, J. E., McCallum, T., & Wetherell, J. (1998). Empirically validated psychological treatments for older adults. *Journal of Mental Health and Aging, 41,* 9–46.

Kendall, P. C., & Chambless, D. L. (Eds.). (1998). Empirically supported psychological therapies [special issue]. *Journal of Consulting and Clinical Psychology, 66*(3), 151–162.

Lonigan, C. J., & Elbert, J. C. (Eds.). (1998). Empirically supported psychosocial interventions for children [special issue]. *Journal of Clinical Child Psychology, 27,* 138–226.

Nathan, P. E., & Gorman, J. M. (Eds.). (1998). *A guide to treatments that work.* New York, NY: Oxford University Press.

Nathan, P. E., & Gorman, J. M. (Eds.). (2002). *A guide to treatments that work* (2nd ed.). New York, NY: Oxford University Press.

Nathan, P. E., & Gorman, J. M. (Eds.). (2007). *A guide to treatments that work* (3rd ed.). New York, NY: Oxford University Press.

Spirito, A. (Ed.). (1999). Empirically supported treatments in pediatric psychology [special issue]. *Journal of Pediatric Psychology, 24,* 87–174.

4

What Are the Identified Empirically Supported Treatments for the Disruptive Behavior Disorders?

Creating an evidence-based psychotherapy treatment plan as described in this series involves integrating those aspects of identified ESTs into each step of the treatment planning process discussed previously. Let's briefly look at efforts to develop and identify ESTs and evidence-based treatment guidelines for disruptive child and adolescent behavior. Recent reviews of the treatment outcome literature for ODD and CD have identified several empirically supported psychological treatments at different levels of empirical support.

Society of Clinical Child and Adolescent Psychology (APA Division 53)

Using the original Division 12 criteria, the Society of Clinical Child and Adolescent Psychology (APA's Division 53) has identified one treatment as well-established and several as probably efficacious.

Empirically Supported Treatment for Disruptive Behavior Disorders

WELL-ESTABLISHED:
- Parent Management Training (PMT), also known as Behavioral Parent Training or Parent Training.

PROBABLY EFFICACIOUS:
- Parent-Child Interaction Therapy
- Problem-Solving Skills Training (also known as Cognitive Problem-Solving Skills Training)
- Anger Control Training
- The Rational-Emotive Mental Health Program

- Group Assertiveness Training
- Multidimensional Treatment Foster Care
- Multisystemic Therapy

PROBABLY EFFICACIOUS MANUALIZED BEHAVIOR MANAGEMENT PROGRAMS:
- Helping the Noncompliant Child
- The enhanced version of the Positive Parenting Program or Triple P
- The Incredible Years program

From the Society of Clinical Child and Adolescent Psychology (APA Division 53).

Kazdin Review

Alan Kazdin, the John M. Musser Professor of Psychology at Yale University and Director of Yale's Parenting Center and Child Conduct Clinic, reviewed treatments specific to conduct disorder (CD) for the latest version of Nathan and Gorman's series, *A Guide to Treatments that Work* (Nathan & Gorman, 2007). He identified several therapies that met the guide's criteria for empirical support, which values well-conducted, replicated, randomized clinical trials. Many of these therapies overlap with those identified by Division 53, whose review included ODD in addition to CD.

Empirically Supported Treatments for Conduct Disorder

- Parent Management Training
- Problem-Solving Skills Training
- Anger Control Training
- Multidimensional Treatment Foster Care
- Multisystemic Therapy
- Functional Family Therapy
- Brief Strategic Family Therapy

From "Psychological Treatments for Conduct Disorder in Children and Adolescents," by A. E. Kazdin, 2007. In P. E. Nathan & J. M. Gorman (Eds.), *A Guide to Treatments That Work* (pp. 71–104). New York, NY: Oxford University Press.

The National Institute for Health and Clinical Excellence (NICE)

Evidence-based practice guidelines published by NICE in Great Britain, which emphasize the highest available levels of evidence, recommend the first-line use of parent management training for disruptive child behavior.

Empirically Supported Treatments for Disruptive Child and Adolescent Behavior

Let's take a quick look at APA's Division 53 empirically supported approaches to treating disruptive child and adolescent behavior.

Parent Management Training (PMT)

- PMT uses social learning principles and practices to alter the pattern of interactions between parent and child so that prosocial behavior is positively reinforced and supported within the family system.
- Through the therapy, parents are taught how to conceptualize, identify, and monitor their child's behavior, how to reinforce prosocial behavior, and how to ignore or set limits on problematic behavior. Through the course of therapy these skills are refined, reinforced, and generalized.
- Home visits and school interventions may also be incorporated.
- Developers of PMT have noted that, in general, the therapy has proven more effective with younger children (typically under 8 years old) than with older children and adolescents.

Parent–Child Interaction Therapy (PCIT)

- PCIT works with parents and younger children, typically aged 2 to 7. As its name suggests, PCIT works with parents and children while they interact to improve the quality of the parent–child relationship.
- Drawing on attachment theory, play therapy, and social learning theory, PCIT emphasizes two primary types of interactions:
  - Child-directed interaction (CDI) in which parents engage their child in a play situation that the child directs, and
  - Parent-directed interaction (PDI) which resembles parent management training in that parents are taught how to use specific behavior management techniques as they play with their child.

Problem-Solving Skills Training (PSST)

- PSST teaches children how to approach conflicts using interpersonal problem-solving skills.
- The therapy employs several techniques such as instruction, modeling, role-playing, feedback, and practice to teach children how to manage interpersonal conflicts.
- It helps children understand their own thought processes and how thoughts influence emotional and behavioral reactions.
- Children are taught how to use a step-by-step approach to solving problems in an adaptive, prosocial manner.
- The treatment uses structured tasks involving games, stories, and other activities to develop these skills, which are then carried into real-life situations.
- Empirical studies of PSST suggest that it is more effective with older children and adolescents than with younger children.

Anger Control Training (ACT)

- Treatment programs classified under anger control training teach children anger management skills, such as how to calm oneself and how to use nonaggressive communication to resolve conflict, as well as using components of parent management training and problem-solving skills training.
- Teacher in-service meetings and consultations, as well as a video-assisted form of role-playing have been used in some recent applications.
- The original version of this treatment, called the Anger Coping Program, was studied as a school-based intervention for older elementary school-aged children identified as aggressive.

Rational Emotive Mental Health Program (REMH)

- REMH is another school-based intervention for 11th and 12th graders with disruptive behavior problems.
- Based on rational emotive therapy (RET), students involved in this intervention participate in daily, 45-minute small group sessions for 12 consecutive weeks.
- Consistent with RET, activities include cognitive restructuring through rational appraisal, role-playing, group-directed discussion, and therapy "homework" assignments.

Group Assertiveness Training

- Group assertiveness training is a well-known intervention that teaches participants how to communicate their thoughts and feelings in a direct, honest, and constructive manner while respecting the rights of others to do the same.
- Resolution of conflict through assertive communication, in the absence of unassertive or aggressive communication, is a primary goal of assertiveness applications to anger management.
- Techniques used include modeling, behavior rehearsal, videotape feedback, and positive reinforcement.

Functional Family Therapy (FFT)

- FFT is an integrative family-based therapy that draws from behavioral, cognitive, and system theories. It analyzes problematic interactions based on the functions they serve in the family system and for the individuals comprising it. The therapy targets change in these interactions to support more adaptive functioning.
- The therapy progresses through three general phases: engagement and motivation, specific behavior change, and generalization (generalization refers to increasing the family's ability to expand and sustain the changes they made during therapy).
- Family systems and social learning interventions are largely used to facilitate these changes.

Brief Strategic Family Therapy (BSFT)

- BSFT was developed through studies of children and families from Hispanic backgrounds. This approach uses family systems approaches while integrating the culturally consistent values of strong family cohesion, parental control, and communication.
- The therapist challenges interaction patterns, facilitates development of alternatives that improve communication, and encourages adoption of the alternatives by family members.
- The development of BSFT is unique in studying cultural features of families and integrating those into the therapy.
- The program has been extended to African American families and has been advanced as a model for developing culturally relevant and sensitive treatments.

Multidimensional Treatment Foster Care (MTFC)

- MTFC is a community-based treatment program that began as an alternative to institutional, residential, and group-care placement of youths with severe and chronic delinquency and has subsequently been applied to children and adolescents referred from mental health or child welfare systems.

- Treatment takes place in the foster home setting, where a treatment team provides intensive supervision, family and individual therapy, skill development, academic support, case management, and medication if needed.

- Foster parents are trained to use Parent Management Training, or PMT, techniques in the foster home setting. Parents or the aftercare resource also undergo PMT. The child is then returned to his or her parents at home.

- The goal is to establish positive prosocial behavior in the child within in a safe, consistent, and positive environment and then transfer the child to a home environment designed to maintain those changes.

Multisystemic Therapy (MST)

- MST was developed to address several limitations of existing mental health services for serious child and adolescent disruptive behavior problems, delinquency, and substance abuse.

- MST conceptualizes youth antisocial behavior as multidetermined and influenced by characteristics of the youth, his or her family, peer group, school, and community contexts.

- It is a pragmatic and goal-oriented treatment that specifically targets those factors in each youth's social network that are contributing to his or her antisocial behavior and/or substance abuse.

- Common objectives for MST include:
  - Improving caregiver discipline practices
  - Enhancing family affective relations
  - Decreasing youth association with deviant peers and increasing youth association with prosocial peers
  - Improving youth school or vocational performance
  - Engaging youth in prosocial recreational outlets
  - Developing an indigenous support network of extended family, neighbors, and friends, to help caregivers achieve and maintain such changes

(*continued*)

- Specific treatment techniques used to facilitate these objectives include cognitive behavioral, behavioral, and the pragmatic family therapies. MST services are delivered in the natural environment (e.g., home, school, community).
- The treatment plan is designed in collaboration with family members and is, therefore, family-driven rather than therapist-driven.
- The ultimate goal of MST is to empower families to build an environment, through the mobilization of indigenous child, family, and community resources that promotes health.

Key Points

COMMON THEMES IN EMPIRICALLY SUPPORTED TREATMENTS FOR DISRUPTIVE BEHAVIOR

1. Working with parents or parents and younger children to train parenting skills that promote prosocial behavior and better interactions using social learning principles.
2. Working with older children and adolescents to build adaptive interactional skills such as problem-solving, anger management, and communication skills.
3. Working with families to improve communication and interactions.
4. Combining these approaches while invoking community systems that will support them for more severely disruptive behavior in adolescents.

Chapter Review

1. Name APA's Division 53 ESTs for disruptive behavior described in the chapter.
2. Briefly describe each APA's Division 53 ESTs for disruptive behavior.
3. What are common themes in ESTs for disruptive behavior?

Chapter Review Test Questions

1. Empirically supported treatments for oppositional and defiant behavior in younger children (age 8 or younger) typically emphasize which of the following?
   A. Teaching the child anger management skills
   B. Teaching the child problem-solving skills
   C. Training parents in child management skills
   D. Training peers who then help the child

2. Which of the following therapeutic approaches identified by APA's Division 53 meets the criteria for a well-established EST?

    A. Anger control training

    B. Assertiveness training

    C. Problem-solving skills training

    D. Parent management training

Selected Chapter References

Reviews of Evidence–Based Treatments

Eyberg, S. M., Nelson, M. M., & Boggs, S. R. (2008). Evidence-based psychosocial treatments for children and adolescents with disruptive behavior. *Journal of Clinical Child and Adolescent Psychology, 37*(1), 215–237.

Kazdin, A. E. (2007). Psychosocial treatments for conduct disorder in children and adolescents. In P. E. Nathan & J. M. Gorman (Eds.), *A guide to treatments that work* (3rd ed., pp. 71–104). New York, NY: Oxford University Press.

Kazdin, A. E., & Weisz, J. R. (Eds.). (2003). *Evidence-based psychotherapies for children and adolescents.* New York, NY: Guilford Press.

Kendall, P. C. (Ed.). (2006). *Child and adolescent therapy: Cognitive-behavioral procedures* (3rd ed.). New York, NY: Guilford Press.

Weisz, J. R., & Kazdin, A. E. (2010). *Evidence-based psychotherapies for children and adolescents* (2nd ed.). New York, NY: Guilford Press.

Empirical Support for Parent Management Training

Bernal, M. E., Klinnert, M. D., & Schultz, L. A. (1980). Outcome evaluation of behavioral parent training and client-centered parent counseling for children with conduct problems. *Journal of Applied Behavior Analysis, 13*, 677–691.

Christensen, A., Johnson, S. M., Phillips, S., & Glasgow, R. E. (1980). Cost effectiveness in behavioral family therapy. *Behavior Therapy, 11*, 208–226.

Forehand, R., & Long, N. (1988). Outpatient treatment of the acting out child: Procedures, long-term follow-up data, and clinical problems. *Advances in Behaviour Research and Therapy, 10*, 129–177.

Hughes, R. C., & Wilson, P. H. (1988). Behavioral parent training: Contingency management versus communication skills training with or without the participation of the child. *Child and Family Behavior Therapy, 10*, 11–23.

Kazdin, A. E. (2005). *Parent management training: Treatment for oppositional, aggressive, and antisocial behavior in children and adolescents.* New York, NY: Oxford University Press.

Kutcher, S., Aman, M., Brooks, S. J., Buitelaar, J., van Daalen, E., Fegert, J., . . . Tyano, S. (2004). International consensus statement on attention-deficit/hyperactivity disorder (ADHD) and disruptive behaviour disorders (DBDs): Clinical implications and treatment practice suggestions. *European Neuropsychopharmacology, 14*, 11–28.

Long, P., Forehand, R., Wierson, M., & Morgan, A. (1994). Does parent training with young noncompliant children have long-term effects? *Behaviour Research and Therapy, 32*, 101-107.

Patterson, G. R., Chamberlain, P., & Reid, J. B. (1982). A comparative evaluation of a parent-training program. *Behavior Therapy, 13*, 638–650.

Clinical Resources

Barkley, R. A. (1997). *Defiant children: A clinician's manual for parent training* (2nd ed.). New York, NY: Guilford Press.

Barkley, R. A., Edwards, G. H., & Robin, A. L. (1999). *Defiant teens: A clinician's manual for assessment and family intervention.* New York, NY: Guilford Press.

Cavell, T. A. (2000). *Working with aggressive children: A practitioner's guide.* Washington, DC: American Psychological Association.

Durand, V. M., & Hieneman, M. (2008). *Helping parents with challenging children: Positive family intervention (facilitator's guide).* New York, NY: Oxford University Press.

Forehand, R., & McMahon, R. J. (1981). *Helping the noncompliant child: A clinician's guide to parent training.* New York, NY: Guilford Press.

Forgatch, M. S., & Patterson, G. R. (2010). Parent management training—Oregon model: An intervention for antisocial behavior in children and adolescents. In J. R. Weisz & A. E. Kazdin (Eds.), *Evidence-based psychotherapies for children and adolescents* (2nd ed., pp. 159–168). New York, NY: Guilford Press.

McMahon, R. J., & Forehand, R. (2005). *Helping the noncompliant child: Family-based treatment for oppositional behavior* (2nd ed.). New York, NY: Guilford Press.

Patterson, G. R. (1976). *Living with children: New methods for parents and teachers* (rev. ed.). Champaign, IL: Research Press.

Patterson, G. R., Reid, J. B., Jones, R. R., & Conger, R. E. (1975). *A social learning approach to family intervention: Families with aggressive children* (Vol. 1). Eugene, OR: Castalia.

Webster-Stratton, C. (2000). *How to promote social and academic competence in young children.* London, UK: Sage.

For more information on empirical support, clinical resources, and parent management training opportunities, visit the Yale Parenting Center and Child Conduct Clinic at: www.yale.edu/childconductclinic/index.html.

Empirical Support for Parent–Child Interaction Therapy

Brestan, E. V., & Eyberg, S. M. (1998). Effective psychosocial treatments of conduct-disordered children and adolescents: 29 years, 82 studies, and 5,272 kids. *Journal of Clinical Child Psychology, 27*, 180–189.

Hood, K. K., & Eyberg, S. M. (2003). Outcomes of parent-child interaction therapy: Mothers' reports on maintenance three to six years after treatment. *Journal of Clinical Child and Adolescent Psychology, 32*, 419–429.

Nixon, R. D., Sweeney, L., Erickson, D. B., & Touyz, S. W. (2003). Parent-child interaction therapy: A comparison of standard and abbreviated treatments for oppositional defiant preschoolers. *Journal of Consulting and Clinical Psychology, 71*, 251–260.

Schuhmann, E. M., Foote, R. C., Eyberg, S. M., Boggs, S. R., & Algina, J. (1998). Efficacy of parent-child interaction therapy: Interim report of a randomized trial with short-term maintenance. *Journal of Clinical Child Psychology, 27*, 34–45.

Zisser, A., & Eyberg, S.M. (2010). Treating oppositional behavior in children using parent-child interaction therapy. In A. E. Kazdin & J. R. Weisz (Eds.), *Evidence-based psychotherapies for children and adolescents* (2nd ed., pp. 179–193). New York, NY: Guilford Press.

Clinical Resources

Brinkmeyer, M., & Eyberg, S. M. (2010). Parent-child interaction therapy for oppositional children. In J. R. Weisz & A. E. Kazdin (Eds.), *Evidence-based psychotherapies for children and adolescents* (2nd ed., pp. 179–193). New York, NY: Guilford Press.

McNeil, C. B., & Humbree-Kigin, T. L. (2010). *Parent-child interaction therapy* (2nd ed.). New York, NY: Springer.

For more information on empirical support, clinical resources, and training opportunities, visit the PCIT Web site at: http://pcit.phhp.ufl.edu/.

Empirical Support for Problem–Solving Skills Training

Baer, R. A., & Nietzel, M. T. (1991). Cognitive and behavioral treatment of impulsivity in children: A meta-analytic review of the outcome literature. *Journal of Clinical Child Psychology, 20*, 400–412.

Durlak, J. A., Fuhrman, T., & Lampman, C. (1991). Effectiveness of cognitive-behavioral therapy for maladapting children: A meta-analysis. *Psychological Bulletin, 110*, 204–214.

Kazdin, A. E., Bass, D., Siegel, T. C., & Thomas, C. (1989). Cognitive behavior therapy and relationship therapy in the treatment of children referred for antisocial behavior. *Journal of Consulting and Clinical Psychology, 57*, 522–536.

Kazdin, A. E., Esveldt-Dawson, K., French, N. H., & Unis, A. S. (1987a). Effects of parent management training and problem-solving skills training combined in the treatment of antisocial child behavior. *Journal of the American Academy of Child & Adolescent Psychiatry, 26,* 416–424.

Kazdin, A. E., Esveldt-Dawson, K., French, N. H., & Unis, A. S. (1987b). Problem-solving skills training and relationship therapy in the treatment of antisocial behavior. *Journal of Consulting and Clinical Psychology, 55,* 76–85.

Kazdin, A. E., Siegel, T. C., & Bass, D. (1992). Cognitive problem-solving skills training and parent management training in the treatment of antisocial behavior in children. *Journal of Consulting and Clinical Psychology, 60,* 733–747.

Kazdin, A. E., & Wassell, G. (2000). Therapeutic changes in children, parents, and families resulting from treatment of children with conduct problems. *Journal of the American Academy of Child and Adolescent Psychiatry, 39,* 414–420.

Sukhodolsky, D. G., Kassinove, H., & Gorman, B. S. (2004). Cognitive-behavioral therapy for anger in children and adolescents: A meta-analysis. *Aggression and Violent Behavior, 9,* 247–269.

Clinical Resources

Barkley, R. A. (1997). *Defiant children: A clinician's manual for assessment and parent training* (2nd ed.). New York, NY: Guilford Press.

Bourke, M. L., & Van Hasselt, V. B. (2001). Social problem-solving skills training for incarcerated offenders: A treatment manual. *Behavioral Modification, 25,* 163–188.

Feindler, E. L., & Ecton, R. B. (1986). *Adolescent anger control: Cognitive-behavioral techniques.* Elmsford, New York: Pergamon.

Finch, A. J., Jr., Nelson, W. M., & Ott, E. S. (1993). *Cognitive-behavioral procedures with children and adolescents: A practical guide.* Needham Heights, MA: Allyn and Bacon.

Kazdin, A. E. (2010). Problem-solving skills training and parent management training for conduct disorder. In J. R. Weisz & A. E. Kazdin (Eds.), *Evidence-based psychotherapies for children and adolescents* (2nd ed., pp. 211–226). New York, NY: Guilford Press.

Larson, J., & Lochman, J. E. (2002). *Helping schoolchildren cope with anger: A cognitive-behavioral intervention.* New York, NY: Guilford Press.

Larson, J., & Lochman, J. E. (in press). *Helping schoolchildren cope with anger: A cognitive-behavioral intervention* (2nd ed.). New York, NY: Guilford Press.

McGuire, J. (2000). *Think first: Outline programme manual case manager's manual and supplements.* London, UK: Home Office Communications Unit.

Shure, M. B. (1992). *I Can Problem Solve (ICPS): An interpersonal cognitive problem solving program.* Champaign, IL: Research Press.

For more information on empirical support, clinical resources, and training opportunities in Problem-Solving Skills Training, visit the Yale Parenting Center and Child Conduct Clinic at: www.yale.edu/childconductclinic/index.html.

Empirical Support for Anger Control Training

Brestan, E. V., & Eyberg, S. M. (1998). Effective psychosocial treatments of conduct-disordered children and adolescents: 29 years, 82 studies, and 5,272 kids. *Journal of Clinical Child Psychology, 27*, 180–189.

Feindler, E. L., & Baker, K. (2004). Current issues in anger management interventions with youth. In A. P. Goldstein, R. Nensen, B. Daleflod, & M. Kalt (Eds.), *New perspectives on aggression replacement training: Practice, research, and application* (pp. 31–50). Hoboken, NJ: Wiley.

Feindler, E. L., Ecton, R. B., Kingsley, D., & Dubey, D. R. (1986). Group anger control training for institutionalized psychiatric male adolescents. *Behavior Therapy, 17*, 109–123.

Feindler, E. L., Marriott, S. A., & Iwata, M. (1984). Group anger control training for junior high school delinquents. *Cognitive Therapy & Research, 8*, 299–311.

Lochman, J. E., Burch, P. P., Curry, J. F., & Lampron, L. B. (1984). Treatment and generalization effects of cognitive-behavioral goal setting interventions with aggressive boys. *Journal of Consulting and Clinical Psychology, 52*, 915–916.

Lochman, J. E., Coie, J. D., Underwood, M. K., & Terry, R. (1993). Effectiveness of a social relations intervention program for aggressive and nonaggressive, rejected children. *Journal of Consulting and Clinical Psychology, 61*, 1053–1058.

Robinson, T. R., Smith, S. W., & Miller, M. D. (2002). Effect of a cognitive-behavioral intervention on responses to anger by middle school students with chronic behavior problems. *Behavioral Disorders, 27*, 256–271.

Sukhodolsky, D. G., Golub, A., Stone, E. C., & Orban, L. (2005). Dismantling anger control training for children: A randomized pilot study of social problem-solving versus social skills training components. *Behavior Therapy, 36*, 15–23.

Sukhodolsky, D. G., Solomon, R. M., & Perine, J. (2000). Cognitive-behavioral anger-control intervention for elementary school children: A treatment-outcome study. *Journal of Child and Adolescent Group Therapy, 10*, 159–170.

Clinical Resources

Barry, T. D., & Pardini, D. A. (2003). Anger control training for aggressive youth. In A. E. Kazdin & J. R. Weisz, (Eds.), *Evidence-based psychotherapies for children and adolescents* (pp. 263–281). New York, NY: Guilford Press.

Feindler, E. L. (1995). An ideal treatment package for children and adolescents with anger disorders. In H. Kassinove (Ed.), *Anger Disorders: Definition, diagnosis, and treatment* (pp. 173–194). New York, NY: Taylor & Francis.

Larson, J. (2005). *Think first: Addressing aggressive behavior in secondary schools.* New York, NY: Guilford Press.

Larson, J., & Lochman, J. E. (2002). *Helping schoolchildren cope with anger: A cognitive-behavioral intervention.* New York, NY: Guilford Press

Larson, J., & Lochman, J. E. (in press). *Helping schoolchildren cope with anger: A cognitive-behavioral intervention* (2nd ed.). New York, NY: Guilford Press.

Lochman, J. E., Boxmeyer, C. L., Powell, N. P., Barry, T. D., & Pardini, D. A. (2010). Anger control training for aggressive youths. In A. E. Kazdin & J. R. Weisz, (Eds.), *Evidence-based psychotherapies for children and adolescents* (2nd ed., pp. 227–242). New York, NY: Guilford Press.

Lochman, J. E., Powell, N. R., Whidby, J. M., & FitzGerald, D. P. (2006). Aggressive children: Cognitive-behavioral assessment and treatment. In P. C. Kendall (Ed.), *Child and adolescent therapy: Cognitive-behavioral procedures* (3rd ed., pp. 33–81). New York, NY: Guilford Press.

For more information, see the anger control training program at: www .therapeuticresources.com/86-22text.html.

See http://bama.ua.edu/~lochman/index2.htm for information on the Coping Power Program, a school-based intervention delivered to at-risk children in the late elementary school and early middle school years, based on an empirical model of risk factors for substance use and delinquency.

Empirical Support for the Rational Emotive Mental Health Program

Block, J. (1978). Effects of a rational-emotive mental health program on poorly achieving, disruptive high school students. *Journal of Counseling Psychology, 25,* 61–65.

DiGiuseppe, R. A., & Bernard, M. E. (1990). The application of rational-emotive theory and therapy to school-aged children. *School Psychology Review, 19,* 268–286.

Watter, D. N. (1988). Rational-emotive education: A review of the literature. *Journal of Rational-Emotive & Cognitive Behavior Therapy, 6,* 139–145.

Clinical Resources

Knaus, W. J. (1977). Rational-emotive education. In A. Ellis & R. Greiger (Eds.), *Handbook of rational-emotive therapy* (pp. 398–408). New York, NY: Springer.

For more information on empirical support, clinical resources, and training opportunities in rational emotive therapy and education, visit http://www.rebtnetwork .org/ and http://rebtnetwork.org/essays/essay.html

Empirical Support for Group Assertiveness Training

Huey, W. C., & Rank, R. C. (1984). Effects of counselor and peer-led group assertive training on black-adolescent aggression. *Journal of Counseling Psychology, 31,* 95–98.

Lee, D. Y., Hallberg, E. T., & Hassard, H. (1979). Effects of assertion training on aggressive behavior of adolescents. *Journal of Counseling Psychology, 26,* 459–461.

Winship, B, J., & Kelley, J. D. (1976). A verbal response model of assertiveness. *Journal of Counseling Psychology, 23,* 215–220.

Clinical Resources

Alberti, R. E., & Emmons, M. L. (2008). *Your perfect right: Assertiveness and equality in your life and relationships* (9th ed.). Atascadero, CA: Impact Publishers.

Empirical Support for Functional Family Therapy

Alexander, J. F., Holtzworth-Munroe, A., & Jameson, P. B. (1994). The process and outcome of marital and family therapy research: Review and evaluation. In A. E. Bergin & S. L. Garfield (Eds.), *Handbook of psychotherapy and behavior change* (4th ed., pp. 595–630). New York, NY: Wiley.

Gordon, D. A., Graves, K., & Arbuthnot, J. (1995). The effect of functional family therapy for delinquents on adult criminal behavior. *Criminal Justice and Behavior, 22,* 60–73.

Clinical Resources

Alexander, J. F., & Parsons, B. V. (1982). *Functional family therapy.* Monterey, CA: Brooks/Cole.

Sexton, T. L., & Alexander, J. F. (1999). *Functional family therapy: Principles of clinical intervention, assessment, and implementation.* Henderson, NV: RCH Enterprises.

For more information on functional family therapy, visit http://www.fftinc.com/index.html.

Empirical Support for Brief Strategic Family Therapy

Coatsworth, J. D., Szapocznik, J., Kurtines, W., & Santisteban, D. A. (1997). Culturally competent psychosocial interventions with antisocial problem behavior in Hispanic youths. In D. M. Stoff, J. Breiling, & J. D. Maser (Eds.), *Handbook of antisocial behavior* (pp. 395–404). New York, NY: Wiley.

Muir, J. A., Schwartz, S. J., & Szapocznik, J. (2004). A program of research with Hispanic and African American families: Three decades of intervention development and testing influenced by the changing cultural context of Miami. *Journal of Marital and Family Therapy, 30,* 285–303.

Robbins, M. S., Schwartz, S., & Szapocznik, J. (2004). Structural ecosystems therapy with Hispanic adolescents exhibiting disruptive behavior disorders. In J. R. Ancis (Ed.), *Culturally responsive interventions: Innovative approaches to working with diverse populations* (pp. 71–99). New York, NY: Brunner-Routledge.

Robbins, M. S., Szapocznik, J., Santisteban, D. A., Hervis, O., Mitrani, V. B., & Schwartz, S. (2003). Brief Strategic Family Therapy for Hispanic youth. In A. E. Kazdin & J. R. Weisz (Eds.), *Evidence-based psychotherapies for children and adolescents* (pp. 407–424). New York, NY: Guilford Press.

Santisteban, D. A., Coatsworth, J. D., Perez-Vidal, A., Kurtines, W. M., Schwartz, S. J., LaPerriere, A., & Szapocznik, J. (2003). Efficacy of brief strategic family therapy in modifying Hispanic adolescent behavior problems and substance use. *Journal of Family Psychology, 17,* 121-133.

Szapocznik, J., & Kurtines, W. M. (1989). *Break-throughs in family therapy with drug-abusing problem youth.* New York, NY: Springer.

Clinical Resources

Robbins, M. S., Szapocznik, J., Santisteban, D. A., Hervis, O., Mitrani, V. B., & Schwartz, S. (2003). Brief Strategic Family Therapy for Hispanic youth. In A. E. Kazdin & J. R. Weisz (Eds.), *Evidence-based psychotherapies for children and adolescents* (pp. 407–424). New York, NY: Guilford Press.

Szapocznik, J., & Kurtines, W. M. (1989). *Break-throughs in family therapy with drug-abusing problem youth.* New York, NY: Springer.

Empirical Support for Multidimensional Treatment Foster Care

Chamberlain, P., & Reid, J. B. (1998). Comparison of two community alternatives to incarceration for chronic juvenile offenders. *Journal of Consulting and Clinical Psychology, 66,* 624–633.

Eddy, J. M., Bridges-Whaley, R., & Chamberlain, P. (2004). The prevention of violent behavior by chronic and serious male juvenile offenders: A 2-year follow-up of a randomized clinical trial. *Journal of Emotional and Behavioral Disorders, 12,* 2–8.

Eddy, J. M., & Chamberlain, P. (2001). Family management and deviant peer association as mediators of the impact of treatment condition on youth antisocial behavior. *Journal of Consulting and Clinical Psychology, 68,* 857–863.

Clinical Resources

Chamberlain, P., Fisher, P. A., & Moore, K. (2002). Multidimensional treatment foster care: Application of the OSLC intervention model to high-risk youth and their families. In J. B. Reid, G. R. Patterson, & J. Snyder (Eds.), *Antisocial behavior in children and adolescents: A developmental analysis and model for intervention* (pp. 203–218). Washington, DC: American Psychological Association.

Smith, D. K., & Chamberlain, P. (2010). Multidimensional treatment foster care for adolescents. In J. R. Weisz & A. E. Kazdin (Eds.), *Evidence-based psychotherapies for children and adolescents* (2nd ed., pp. 243–258). New York, NY: Guilford Press.

For more information on multidimensional treatment foster care, visit the Web site, at www.mtfc.com.

Empirical Support for Multisystemic Therapy

Borduin, C. M., Mann, B. J., Cone, L. T., Henggeler, S. W., Fucci, B. R., Blaske, D. M., & Williams, R. A. (1995). Multisystemic treatment of serious juvenile offenders: Long-term prevention of criminality and violence. *Journal of Consulting and Clinical Psychology, 63*, 569–578.

Henggeler, S. W., Melton, G. B., Brondino, M. J., Scherer, D. G., & Hanley, J. H. (1997). Multisystemic therapy with violent and chronic juvenile offenders and their families: The role of treatment fidelity in successful dissemination. *Journal of Consulting and Clinical Psychology, 65*, 821–833.

Henggeler, S. W., Melton, G. B., & Smith, L. A. (1992). Family preservation using multisystemic therapy: An effective alternative to incarcerating serious juvenile offenders. *Journal of Consulting and Clinical Psychology, 60*, 953–961.

Henggeler, S. W., Pickrel, S. G., & Brondino, M. J. (1999). Multisystemic treatment of substance-abusing and -dependent delinquents: Outcomes, treatment fidelity, and transportability. *Mental Health Services Research, 1*, 171–184.

Henggeler, S. W., Schoenwald, S. K., Borduin, C. M., Rowland, M. D., & Cunningham, P. B. (1998). *Multisystemic treatment of antisocial behavior in children and adolescents.* New York: Guilford Press.

Scherer, D. G., Brondino, M. J., Henggeler, S. W., Melton, G. B., & Hanley, J. H. (1994). Multisystemic family preservation therapy: Preliminary findings from a study of rural and minority serious adolescent offenders. *Journal of Emotional and Behavioral Disorders, 2*, 198–206.

Clinical Resources

Henggeler, S. W., & Schaffer, C. (2010). Treating serious antisocial behavior using multisystemic therapy. In J. Weisz & A. Kazdin (Eds.), *Evidence-based psychotherapies for children and adolescents* (2nd ed., pp. 259-276). New York, NY: Guilford Press.

Henggeler, S. W., Schoenwald, S. K., Borduin, C. M., Rowland, M. D., & Cunningham, P. B. (1998). *Multisystemic treatment of antisocial behavior in children and adolescents.* New York, NY: Guilford Press.

Henggeler, S. W., Schoenwald, S. K., Rowland, M. D., & Cunningham, P. B. (2002). *Serious emotional disturbance in children and adolescents: Multisystemic therapy.* New York, NY: Guilford Press.

For more information on empirical support, clinical resources, and training opportunities in multisystemic therapy, visit the Web site at: www.mstservices.com.

Empirical Support for the Incredible Years Program

Reid, M. J., Webster-Stratton, C., & Hammond, M. (2003). Follow-up of children who received the Incredible Years intervention for oppositional defiant disorder: Maintenance and prediction of 2-year outcome, *Behavior Therapy, 34,* 471–491.

Webster-Stratton, C. (1984). Randomized trial of two parent-training programs for families with conduct-disordered children. *Journal of Consulting and Clinical Psychology, 52,* 666–678.

Webster-Stratton, C., & Hammond, M. (1997). Treating children with early-onset conduct problems: A comparison of child and parent training interventions. *Journal of Consulting and Clinical Psychology, 65,* 93–109.

Webster-Stratton, C., Reid, M., & Hammond, M. (2001). Social skills and problem-solving training for children with early-onset conduct problems: Who benefits? *Journal of Child Psychology and Psychiatry, 42,* 943–952.

Webster-Stratton, C., Reid, M., & Hammond, M. (2004). Treating children with early-onset conduct problems: Intervention outcomes for parent, child, and teacher training. *Journal of Clinical Child and Adolescent Psychology, 33,* 105–124.

Clinical Resources

Webster-Stratton, C. (2000). *How to promote social and academic competence in young children.* London, UK: Sage.

Webster-Stratton, C., & Reid, M. J. (2010). The Incredible Years parents, teachers, and children training series: A multifaceted treatment approach for young children. In J. Weisz & A. Kazdin (Eds.), *Evidence-based psychotherapies for children and adolescents* (2nd ed., pp. 194–210). New York, NY: Guilford Press.

For more information on empirical support, clinical resources, and training opportunities, visit the Incredible Years Web site at: www.incredibleyears.com/.

Empirical Support for Positive Parenting Program (Triple P)

Bor, W., Sanders, M. R., & Markie-Dadds, C. (2002). The effects of the Triple P-positive parenting program on preschool children with co-occurring disruptive behavior and attentional-hyperactive difficulties. *Journal of Abnormal Child Psychology, 30,* 571–587.

Sanders, M. R., Markie-Dadds, C., Tully, L. A., & Bor, W. (2000). The Triple P-positive parenting program: A comparison of enhanced, standard, and self-directed behavioral family intervention for parents of children with early onset conduct problems. *Journal of Consulting and Clinical Psychology, 68,* 624–640.

Clinical Resources

For information on empirical support, clinical resources, and training opportunities visit the Triple P Web site at: www.triplep.net/.

Empirical Support for Helping the Noncompliant Child

Peed, S., Roberts, M., & Forehand, R. (1977). Evaluation of the effectiveness of a standardized parent training program in altering the interaction of mothers and their noncompliant children. *Behavior Modification, 1,* 323–350.

Wells, K. C., & Egan, J. (1988). Social learning and systems family therapy for childhood oppositional disorder: Comparative treatment outcome. *Comprehensive Psychiatry, 29,* 138–146.

Clinical Resources

Forehand, R., & McMahon, R. J. (1981). *Helping the noncompliant child: A clinician's guide to parent training.* New York, NY: Guilford Press.

McMahon, R. J., & Forehand, R. (2005). *Helping the noncompliant child: Family-based treatment for oppositional behavior* (2nd ed.). New York, NY: Guilford Press.

For more information and resources visit: www.strengtheningfamilies.org/html/programs_1999/02_HNCC.html.

Bibliotherapy Resources

Durand, V. M., & Hieneman, M. (2008). *Helping parents with challenging children: Positive family intervention (parent's workbook).* New York, NY: Oxford University Press.

Forehand, R., & Long, N. (1996). *Parenting the strong-willed child.* Chicago, IL: Contemporary Books.

Forehand, R., & Long, N. (2002). *Parenting the strong-willed child: The clinically proven five-week program for parents of two- to six-year-olds* (rev. ed.). Chicago, IL: Contemporary Books.

Kazdin, A. E. (2009). *The Kazdin method for parenting the defiant child: With no pills, no therapy, no contest of wills.* New York, NY: Mariner.

Patterson, G. R. (1975). *Families: Applications of social learning to family life.* Champaign, IL: Research Press.

Patterson, G. R. (1977). *Living with children: New methods for parents and teachers.* Champaign, IL: Research Press.

Shure, M. B. (1996). *Raising a thinking child: Help your young child to resolve everyday conflicts and get along with others.* New York, NY: Pocket Books.

For information on training opportunities in many of the empirically supported treatments discussed in this program, visit Strengthening America's Families at www.strengtheningfamilies.org/.

5

How Do You Integrate Empirically Supported Treatments Into Treatment Planning?

Construction of an empirically informed treatment plan for disruptive child and adolescent behavior involves integrating objectives and treatment interventions consistent with identified empirically supported treatments (ESTs) into a client's treatment plan after you have determined that the client's primary problem fits those described in the target population of the EST research. As noted earlier, we focus in this DVD on disruptive behavior of the oppositional defiant disorder (ODD) and conduct disorder (CD) type. Of course, implementing ESTs must be done in consideration of important client, therapist, and therapeutic relationship factors—consistent with the APA's definition of evidence-based practice.

Definitions

The behavioral definition statements describe *how the problem manifests itself in the client*. Although there are several common features of ODD and CD, the behavioral definition of disruptive behavior for your client will be unique and specific to him or her. Your assessment will need to identify which features best characterize your client's presentation. Accordingly, the *behavioral definition* of your treatment plan is tailored to your individual client's clinical picture. When the primary problem reflects a recognized psychiatric diagnosis, the behavioral definition statements are usually closely aligned with diagnostic criteria such as those provided in the DSM or ICD.

Since disruptive behavior can be related to a diagnosis of oppositional defiant disorder (ODD) or conduct disorder (CD), we present the behavioral definitions for both conditions here. Although there is overlap in the definition statements for ODD and CD, it is evident that the statements for CD reflect a more serious pathology. Children who are the concern of parents who present for therapy often do not meet all the criteria for ODD or certainly not CD. In these cases a diagnosis of disruptive behavior disorder (NOS) may be used. The treatment plan should be tailored to each client's unique expression of disruptive behavior.

Examples of common ODD definition statements are the following:

➤ Has a history of explosive, aggressive outbursts
➤ Often argues with authority figures over requests or rules
➤ Deliberately annoys people as a means of gaining control
➤ Blames others rather than accept responsibility for own problems
➤ Displays angry overreaction to perceived disapproval, rejection, or criticism
➤ Has a persistent pattern of challenging, resenting, or disrespecting authority figures
➤ Demonstrates body language of tense muscles (e.g., clenched fists or jaw, glaring looks, or refusal to make eye contact)
➤ Uses verbally abusive language
➤ Abuses substances to cope with feelings of anger and alienation
➤ Evidences significant impairment in social, academic, or occupational functioning

Examples of common CD definition statements are the following:

➤ Persistent refusal to comply with rules or expectations in the home, school, or community (e.g., breaks curfew, multiple runaways)
➤ Excessive fighting, threatening, and intimidation of others; physical cruelty or violence toward people or animals; and destruction of property through fire setting or other means
➤ History of stealing at home, at school, or in the community, including breaking into property
➤ Has repeatedly been truant from school
➤ Repeated conflict with authority figures at home, at school, or in the community
➤ Impulsivity as manifested by poor judgment, taking inappropriate risks, and failing to stop and think about consequences of actions
➤ Numerous attempts to deceive others through lying, conning, or manipulating
➤ Consistent failure to accept responsibility for misbehavior accompanied by a pattern of blaming others
➤ Verbalizes little or no remorse for misbehavior
➤ Multiple sexual partners, lack of emotional commitment, and engaging in unsafe sexual practices
➤ Has forced someone into sexual activity
➤ Uses mood-altering substances on a regular basis
➤ Evidences significant impairment in social, academic, or occupational functioning

Goals

The next step in treatment planning is to determine long-term goals. Goals are broad statements describing what you and the client would like the result of therapy to be.

One statement may suffice but more than one can be used in the treatment plan. Examples of common goal statements for disruptive behavior are the following:

➤ Comply with rules and expectations in the home, school, and community consistently.
➤ Stop blaming others for problems and accept responsibility for own feelings, thoughts, and behaviors.
➤ Express anger in a controlled, respectful manner on a consistent basis.
➤ Parents learn and implement good child behavioral management skills.
➤ Parents establish and maintain appropriate parent-child boundaries, setting firm, consistent limits when the client acts out in an aggressive or rebellious manner.
➤ Reach a level of reduced tension, increased satisfaction, and improved communication with family and/or other authority figures.
➤ Eliminate all illegal and antisocial behavior.
➤ Terminate all acts of violence or cruelty toward people or animals and stop any destruction of property.
➤ Demonstrate marked improvement in impulse control.

Objectives and Interventions

Objectives are statements that describe *small, observable steps the client must achieve* toward attaining the goal of successful treatment. Intervention statements describe the *actions taken by the therapist* to assist the client or the parents in achieving his/her objectives. Each objective must be paired with at least one intervention.

Assessment

All approaches to quality treatment start with a thorough assessment of the nature and history of the client's presenting problems. EST approaches rely on a thorough psychosocial assessment of the nature, history, and severity of the problem as experienced by the client and his or her parents.

Table 5.1 on the following page contains examples of assessment objectives and interventions for disruptive behavior.

Psychoeducation

A typical feature of many ESTs for disruptive behavior is initial and ongoing psychoeducation. A common emphasis is helping the client or the parents learn about disruptive behavior, the treatment, and its rationale. Often, books or other reading material are recommended to the client to supplement psychoeducation done in session. It is important to instill hope in the client and have him or her on board as a partner in the treatment process. With ESTs, discussing their demonstrated efficacy with the client can facilitate this.

Table 5.1   Assessment Objectives and Interventions

Objectives	Interventions
1. Identify major concerns regarding the child's misbehavior and the associated parenting approaches that have been tried.	1. Conduct a clinical interview focused on pinpointing the nature and severity of the child's misbehavior. 2. Probe as to how the parents have attempted to respond to the child's misbehavior and what triggers and reinforcements may be contributing to the behavior.
2. Describe any conflicts that result from the different approaches to parenting that each partner has.	1. Assess the parent's consistency in their approach to the child and whether they have experienced conflicts between them over how to react to the child.
3. Parents and child cooperate with psychological assessment to further delineate the nature of the presenting problem.	1. Administer psychological instruments designed to objectively assess parent-child relational conflict (e.g., the Parenting Stress Index [PSI], the Parent-Child Relationship Inventory [PCRI], or the Intra and Interpersonal Relations Scale), traits of oppositional defiance or conduct disorder (e.g., Adolescent Psychopathology Scale—Short Form [APS-SF], Millon Adolescent Clinical Inventory [MACI]); give the clients feedback regarding the results of the assessment; readminister as needed to assess outcome. 2. Conduct or arrange for psychological testing to help in assessing whether a comorbid condition (e.g., depression, Attention-Deficit/Hyperactivity Disorder (ADHD) is contributing to disruptive behavior problems; follow up accordingly with client and parents regarding treatment options; readminister as needed to assess outcome.
4. Cooperate with an evaluation for possible treatment with psychotropic medications to assist in anger and behavioral control, and take medications consistently, if prescribed.	1. Assess the client for the need for psychotropic medication to assist in control of anger and other misbehaviors; refer him/her to a physician for an evaluation for prescription medication; monitor prescription compliance, effectiveness, and side effects; provide feedback to the prescribing physician.

COMMON EMPHASES OF INITIAL PSYCHOEDUCATION

- Teaching the client about the nature and etiology of the diagnosed condition
- Informing the client regarding the various treatment options that are consistent with successful research results
- Explaining the rationale behind the treatment approach that will be used
- Utilizing reading assignments as homework, if needed, to facilitate understanding of these psychoeducational goals

Table 5.2 contains examples of psychoeducational objectives and interventions for disruptive behavior.

Table 5.2   Psychoeducational Objectives and Interventions

Objectives	Interventions
5. Verbalize alternative ways to think about and manage anger and misbehavior.	1. Assist the client in reconceptualizing anger as involving different components (cognitive, physiological, affective, and behavioral) that go through predictable phases (e.g., demanding expectations not being met leading to increased arousal and anger leading to acting out) that can be managed. 2. Assist the client in identifying the positive consequences of managing anger and misbehavior (e.g., respect from others and self, cooperation from others, improved physical health, etc.); ask the client to agree to learn new ways to conceptualize and manage anger and misbehavior.
6. Parents verbalize an understanding of parent management training skills.	1. Use a parent management training approach to teach the parents how parent and child behavioral interactions can encourage or discourage positive or negative behavior and that changing key elements of those interactions (e.g., prompting and reinforcing positive behaviors) can be used to promote positive change (e.g., see *Parenting the Strong-Willed Child* by Forehand & Long; *Living with Children* by Patterson). 2. Ask the parents to read parent training manuals (e.g., *Parenting the Strong-Willed Child* by Forehand & Long) or watch and process videotapes demonstrating the techniques being learned in session (see Webster-Stratton, 1994).

Demonstration Vignette

Psychoeducation of Parents

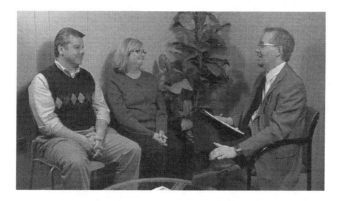

(continued)

Here we present the transcript of the dialogue depicted in the psychoeducation vignette.

Therapist: Last session, we talked about Lou's misbehavior and your frustrations with trying unsuccessfully to get it to change. You talked about the many things you have tried in the past few months and how it has even led to conflict between the two of you as the atmosphere at home has gotten more tense for everyone.

Mom: Yes, it has.

Therapist: Raising a child is a challenge for everyone, and all parents have times when they want to pull their hair out or scream. So you're in good company. No child comes with an instruction book on *How to Raise Me to Become a Well-Behaved Child*. We all struggle with how to do it, so do not be too hard on yourselves. Someone once said that raising kids is like making waffles. You want to throw the first one away because it's always a mess. Poor Lou is your first one and you obviously don't want to throw him away, but you do want him to obey more often, right?

Mom: Absolutely. He's been a challenge for us for a long time, but we love him and we think he's a good kid.

Therapist: Of course he is. I just want you to hear that your parenting struggles are normal. I believe I can help you implement some techniques that will help. It will be important for you to work as a team so there is consistency in the approach to Lou's behavior. Has consistency been an issue between you?

Dad: Yes, it has. Sue tends to be harder on Lou than I am, but she's with him more, so she gets frustrated more often too.

Therapist: That is understandable. It's very common for partners to have different ideas about how to deal with child rearing and discipline. A lot of that has to do with how we were raised ourselves.
          We take that experience into our marriage and into our new family with our own children. Sometimes we imitate how we were raised, and other times we react against how we were raised.
          Either way, our histories shape the pattern we bring to our new family. It's important now for us to agree to work together as we institute some new approaches. Can you commit to that?

Dad: We have to. Our old ones aren't getting the job done. It'll be good to have some outside ideas to follow. I'm ready.

Mom: Me too. We've been at each other's throat at times, but we both know it's best for Lou and the other kids if we work as a team.

Therapist: Perfect. An important perspective for us to keep is that we want to focus on Lou's behavior in particular situations, not more generally on him as child or person. As you said, Lou is a good child. We want to help him adopt some new behaviors in certain situations. A central principal we will be following is that behavior is engaged in by children because it "works" for them. It gets them what they are after, whether they themselves realize it or not. We call this the *reinforcement principal*. Parents provide reinforcement to children's behavior, often without being aware of it, and often in subtle ways. Just the day-to-day interaction in the home sets the stage for the behaviors you are seeing.

We also will be shifting the focus from negative behaviors—or misbehaviors—to prosocial, positive, or desired behavior. Simply stated, we want to catch Lou and the other kids in the family being good and reward that behavior. "Catch them being good" is a key concept.

Mom: I try to do that but it's hard to stick to it when the misbehavior is so frequent.

Therapist: I definitely understand that. We'll need to support each other in trying to be consistent in focusing on good behavior. And we will develop ways to do it in a systematic manner by defining exactly what behavior we want to reward, rewarding it, and then gradually adjusting the rewards to help the behavior become more established.

Dad: I like that idea. We need to be more consistent in focusing on what we want to see Lou do right and hand out rewards for it.

Therapist: Exactly right. And after we have established this practice of "contingency reinforcement," which is giving rewards based on good behavior, then we'll focus on setting limits on undesirable behavior or enforcing consequences like time out, removal of privileges, or adding home chore assignments. But again, we will need to do this in a systematic manner that specifies exactly what behavior is getting a consequence and what the consequence will be. In fact, we will write out our plan for rewards and for negative consequences.

Mom: This isn't going to be easy, is it? Being so specific about behavior and plans to reward it.

Therapist: No, it takes work, good communication, follow-through, and consistency on the parental team.

Mom: Well, we haven't been consistent; I know that.

Therapist: And that again is the norm. One more thing I want to mention. We want to keep in mind that Lou is only 8. So we'll have to tailor our expectations about his behavior to his age and developmental level.

Dad: That's right. I've said this to Sue more than once. She expects too much of him at his age.

Mom: And you treat him like he's a baby.

Therapist: There's going to be disagreement on what to expect from him. That is normal and expected too. So we'll have to work together to set expectations for positive behavior that we can agree on and support. Even then, we may have to adjust our expectations along the way; we may not get it perfect right away. But to get started, I want to give you some reading material on stages of development and typical behaviors to expect. For now, I would like to ask you to gather some data by observing Lou and completing this Child Behavior Checklist. This will give us some idea as to what behaviors we need to focus on first in the coming weeks. Let's take a look at this form together so you understand how to fill it out this week . . .

Critique of the Psychoeducation Demonstration Vignette

The following points were made in the critique:

a. The therapist makes the parents feel comfortable as he relates at their level and normalizes their struggles in parenting without being judgmental.

   b. The need for consistency between parents is stressed, as well as acknowledging how difficult this is.
   c. The therapist rightly points out how focusing on the reinforcement of positive behavior teaches more than punishing negative behavior.
   d. The need to have age-appropriate developmental expectations for the child's behavior is correctly made clear by the therapist.

Additional points that could be made:

   a. I like how the therapist brings out the history that each parent brings to the parenting task from his/her own family of origin—either by seeing parents as a model or as a reaction against their parents' methods. More discussion could have been explored on this issue as to how these experiences have influenced their parenting style with their own children.
   b. The therapist made the point that children engage in behavior that works for them to get rewards. Parents are often reinforcing misbehavior without realizing it. Examples of this would have been helpful to drive the point home. He might have tried eliciting examples of this from the parents with their own child.
   c. The therapist honestly acknowledged that it is going to be hard work to define behavioral expectations precisely and then reinforce these behaviors with consistency.

Comments you would like to make:

_____

_____

_____

_____

   Homework: The homework exercise "Learning to Parent as a Team" (*Adult Psychotherapy Homework Planner*, 2nd ed., by Jongsma) is an example of an intervention consistent with parenting assessment and psychoeducation. It is designed to help the parents describe their own perceived strengths and weaknesses as well as listing ways they could support each other with consistent parenting (see www.wiley.com/go/DBehwb).

Assessment/Psychoeducation Review

   1. What are common emphases of initial psychoeducation?

Assessment/Psychoeducation Review Test Question

1. At what point in therapy is psychoeducation conducted?

   A. At the end of therapy
   B. During the assessment phase
   C. During the initial treatment session
   D. Throughout therapy

Parent Management Training (PMT)

The PMT method uses social learning principles and practices to increase the frequency of desirable child behaviors. Examples include specifying problem behaviors, identifying the influences of parental behavior on that of the child, determining whether the reaction encourages or discourages the behavior, and learning alternative actions to encourage appropriate child behavior.

In parent training, there is an emphasis on establishing realistic age-appropriate rules for acceptable and unacceptable behavior. Parents are assisted in pinpointing target behaviors precisely, agreeing to work together as a team to ignore misbehavior as much as is practical, and reinforce positive behavior—sometimes described as "catching the child being good." They are directed to implement the reinforcement techniques using clearly established target behaviors and stipulated rewards. Homework assignments are used to guide the process of learning and implementation.

Key Points

KEY FEATURES OF PMT

- PMT uses social learning principles and practices to alter the pattern of interactions between parent and child.
- Prosocial behavior is positively reinforced and supported within the family system.
- Parents learn how to conceptualize, identify, and monitor their child's behavior.
- Parents are taught how to reinforce prosocial behavior, and how to ignore or set limits on problematic behavior.
- PMT is particularly effective with younger children (typically under 8 years old).

Table 5.3 contains examples of a PMT objective and interventions for disruptive behavior.

Table 5.3   Parent Management Training Objective and Interventions

Objective	Interventions
7. Parents implement parent management training skills to identify and reinforce a child's desirable behavior.	1. Teach the parents how to specifically define and identify problem behaviors, identify their own reactions to the behavior, determine whether the reaction encourages or discourages the behavior, and generate alternatives to the problem behavior. 2. Assign the parents to implement key parenting practices consistently, including establishing realistic age-appropriate rules for acceptable and unacceptable behavior, prompting of positive behavior in the environment, use of positive reinforcement to encourage behavior (e.g., praise and clearly established rewards), and the use of calm, clear, direct instruction, time out, and other loss-of-privilege practices for problem behavior. 3. Assign the parents home exercises in which they implement and record results of implementation exercises (or assign "Clear Rules, Positive Reinforcement, Appropriate Consequences" in the *Brief Adolescent Therapy Homework Planner*, 2nd ed., by Jongsma, Peterson, & McInnis); review in session, providing corrective feedback toward improved, appropriate, and consistent use of skills.

Demonstration Vignette

Parent Management Training

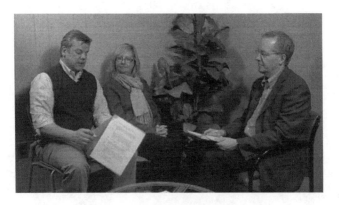

Here we present the transcript of the dialogue depicted in the parent training vignette.

Therapist: Folks, let me just start by summarizing where we are. You started out expressing your concerns and frustrations surrounding Lou's behavior. And then you gathered some observational data about his behavior using the Child Behavior Checklist and the Parent Daily Report I sent home with you over the last couple of weeks.

Parents: Yes, we did.

Therapist: From all of that information, we pinpointed two positive behaviors you would like to see from Lou with increased frequency: First, keeping his bedroom tidy—specifically, putting his clothes away when he takes them off . . . making his bed every morning when he gets up . . . and then secondly, sitting at the dinner table and eating with the rest of the family at suppertime. Finally, you have tracked and charted the frequency of these two behaviors and noted what happened before, during, and after these behaviors occurred. So we have come quite a long way to this point. Sue, is that a fair summary of our work up to today?

Mom: Yes it is. We still haven't made much progress in changing Lou's behavior, and that is frustrating, but we have at least set some clear goals!

Therapist: I hear you about the frustration. To make this work, we have to be prepared before we start to change the behavior in a systematic way.

Dad: And Lou is wondering what is coming next. He sees us marking things down but not doing much else.

Therapist: I'll bet he is curious. Our next step is to use some of the rewards you both listed would hopefully be effective for Lou. We now want to pair the rewards with the two positive behaviors we have pinpointed and measured: clean room and eating supper with the family. What rewards do you think might be most effective, Mark?

Dad: Well, let's see. Here's the list we made a couple of weeks ago. I would say getting his Gameboy back. Another would be getting a pass to play nine holes of golf. He loves playing golf on that par-three course close to home.

Therapist: Perfect choices. Good. Now we need to decide how often Lou must do the behavior in a week's time before he gets the reward. Remember I said earlier that initially he should get the reward at least 75% of the time, or the bar is likely to be set too high. What do you think, Sue?

Mom: I think we could start at 3 times a week and see what happens. Can we raise the level expected later? That would be changing the rules.

Therapist: Oh yes. You need to explain to Lou that the expectations may change over time but this where we are starting.

Dad: He won't be happy about that, but he's not very happy now anyway.

Therapist: He may not, but it's important for him to see that you mean what you say. You can express that you understand he may not be happy, but that can't change the way it's going to be. And remember, he may revolt some now, but if you stay consistent through that he is likely to adapt to it.

Mom: I understand.

(continued)

> Therapist: So let's continue to monitor and chart the two behaviors. Remember also that you are not going to get on his case if he does not do these two things. We want to ignore the negative even if it's difficult, and accentuate the positive by rewarding it as we discussed.
>
> Mom: Are we ever going to set limits on him, or correct his misbehavior?
>
> Therapist: Yes, you can set limits and have some consequences now if his misbehavior is serious, but ideally we want to hold off on instituting that aspect of parenting—like using time out, privilege removal, or adding chores—until we have a good grasp of rewarding the good behavior consistently. As much as possible I recommend that you ignore the negative behavior. As I said before, behavior changes much more quickly when positive behavior gets rewarded or reinforced than when negative behavior gets punished.
>
> Mom: Okay. At least we are working on something constructive now, and we are doing it together, so that feels good to me.
>
> Therapist: Very good. Now let's review. We have two target behaviors and Lou will get his choice of two rewards if he does either of them three times this week. Does that sound right?

Critique of the PMT Demonstration Vignette

The following points were made in the critique:

   a. It is difficult for parents to learn to pinpoint behavior and chart it consistently. Breaking down complex behaviors into specific components to count and reinforce is not easy. Then they need to be strongly motivated to collect data in the assessment phase because they are eager to get to the intervention phase.

   b. The therapist makes a good point about how behavior changes more quickly when positive behavior is rewarded than when negative behavior is punished. This could have been elaborated on and driven home more.

   c. Teaching parents to reward prosocial behavior is an ongoing objective. It is a mind-set of "catching the child being good."

   d. Parent-child interaction therapy would use similar parent training techniques, but apply them while observing the parents and child interact in a play therapy approach.

Additional points that could be made:

   a. The therapist stressed how the parents need to stay in control of the reinforcement program even if the child objects and is unhappy. This is important but not easily done.

b. Ignoring negative behavior while focusing on reinforcing targeted positive behaviors is understandably difficult for parents to accept. You may need to provide a time-out technique earlier to help them manage an out of control child.

Comments you would like to make:

_____

_____

_____

_____

Homework: The homework exercise "Using Reinforcement Principles in Parenting" (*Adult Psychotherapy Homework Planner*, 2nd ed., by Jongsma) is an exercise that teaches the basic tools of behavior modification, how to write clear and precise behavioral goals, and the importance of positive reinforcement in successful parenting (see www.wiley.com/go/DBehwb).

Parent Management Training Review

1. What are the key features of Parent Management Training?

Parent Management Training Review Test Question

1. Which of the following practices is most consistent with Parent Management Training (PMT)?

   A. Identifying and punishing undesirable behavior
   B. Identifying and rewarding desirable behavior
   C. Teaching disruptive children anger management skills
   D. Teaching disruptive children problem-solving skills

Skills Training Approaches (Anger Control/Problem-Solving)

This next set of objectives and interventions reflect skills-training approaches typically used with older children and adolescents. In this example, objectives and interventions consistent with an application of anger control training are presented.

An emphasis in these types of interventions is the development of coping skills that help the client identify when they are getting angry, stop the process, and problem-solve an adaptive solution, sometimes referred to as "stop, think, and act." The focus is not on just teaching these skills one time, but rather on applying them over and over within role-playing sessions to different anger trigger situations in the client's life. Parent management training is often used in concert with skills training approaches. Teacher in-service meetings and consultations, as well as a video-assisted form of role-playing, have been used in some applications.

Key Points

EMPHASES IN ANGER CONTROL/PROBLEM-SOLVING SKILLS TRAINING

- The approach is typically done with older children and adolescents.
- The client learns coping skills that help him or her identify when he or she is getting angry, stop the process, and problem-solve an adaptive solution.
- Skills include anger management, calming, nonaggressive communication skills, and problem-solving.
- Techniques used include instruction, modeling, role-playing, and homework assignments.
- Adjunctive parent management training may be used.
- In-service meetings and consultations with the client's teacher have been used in some applications.

Table 5.4 contains examples of an anger control/problem-solving skills training objective and interventions for disruptive behavior.

Table 5.4   Anger Control/Problem–Solving Skills Training Objective and Interventions

Objective	Interventions
8. Implement anger control training techniques to manage and control anger.	1. Use modeling, role-playing, and behavioral rehearsal to teach the client anger control techniques that include stop, think, and act as well as problem solving skills; role play the application of the skills to multiple situations in the client's life. 2. Assign the client to implement the anger control techniques in his/her daily living; review these incidents and reinforce success and redirect for failure.

Demonstration Vignette

Anger Control/Problem-Solving Skills Training

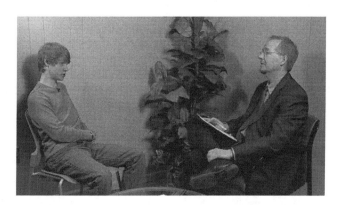

Here we present the transcript of the dialogue depicted in the anger control/problem-solving skills training vignette.

Therapist: Let's look closer at that incident you described when you came home 45 minutes late last night and ended up in a blow-up with your mom, who was waiting up for you.

Client: What about it? She acts like she's a cop or something with all her questions. She's always on my case. I was a little late. It's not a big deal. She doesn't have to grill me.

Therapist: It would have been better if it hadn't been such a big conflict?

Client: Yeah. It didn't have to be such big deal.

Therapist: Well, let's look at ways to approach conflicts that might make them less of a big deal in the future. Why don't we try our role-playing routine with this situation? You know how it goes. You play Mom, and I'll play you. But this time I'm going to try to find a way to respond to this scenario that reduces the chances of it becoming a conflict. What I'm going to do is to use the problem-solving approach we've been talking about. You okay with that?

Client: All right. I guess so.

Therapist: Okay. Just to get some understanding of this, I'd like you to pretend that I just walked in; and you ask me what your Mom asked you when you walked in. What did she say?

Client: "Where have you been? Why are you so late? You know you are supposed to be home at 11:00."

Therapist: Okay, now is this where you started getting angry?

Client: Yeah.

Therapist: Okay. Anger is a real feeling and should be addressed, but instead of increasing the conflict, I'm going use problem-solving. And I'm going to tell you how I'm thinking about it as I do it.

Client: Okay.

(*continued*)

Therapist: So I want to look at what my options are for a response. I want to stop and think before I act. One way to think about it is like they do on a football or basketball replay on TV when they say "Freeze it right there!" to analyze what happened during a play.

Client: Okay, like we did before.

Therapist: Exactly. It's really important that we don't just react quickly to our feelings. We need to step back, take a quick time-out and a deep breath and think about the next step. You can even say to yourself "Time out!" Since we've talked with your folks about our work on problem-solving you can even say to Mom, "Let me think about this a second."

Client: If she would go for that.

Therapist: You might be surprised, and if not we can deal with that.

Client: Okay.

Therapist: All right, so our next step is to look at the possibilities for responding to this trigger situation. Let's get some out there and then see which one looks best. First, you could do what you did, and yell at her about her trying to control your life—like: '"Can't you just get off my back? You're always trying to control everything I do!" Or, you could get angry, ignore her, and walk off to your room. A third is you could stay calm and tell her what actually delayed you getting home on time. For example, you could say, "Sheila was driving and she has a later curfew so she blew me off when I said I better get home when it was 11. I didn't want to push the issue with her and the other girls there." Which of those do you think might get a more positive result than what you ended up with last night?

Client: Well, the last one would be the best. And that's exactly what happened but she doesn't give me a chance to explain. She's firing one question after the other at me, and I just blew up.

Therapist: I understand. It's important to take control of your reactions in these situations. Regardless of what the other person is doing, you have control over your own reactions. But you have to decide to be in control. How do you do this? Stop, take a breath, and think before you act. The results are almost always going to be better. You ask yourself, "What are my choices?" and then "Which choice is going to get the best outcome?" Then choose and act.

Client: That's hard for me.

Therapist: I know it is. That's why we're going to practice this problem-solving approach over and over in many different situations, so it becomes easier and more automatic for you. Let's do the role-reversal thing and have you play yourself and I'll play Mom. This time you try the third option like I did it. Ready?

Client: Okay.

Therapist: "Where have you been, Lou? Why are you so late? You were supposed to be home at 11:00."

Client: "Can I just think about this a second."

Therapist: "Fine."

Client:	"Sheila was driving and she doesn't have to be home so early, so she told me to grow up when I said I need to get home by 11. I didn't want to push it with her when the other girls were around."
Therapist:	"I see. I understand it was hard for you to push it with Sheila. I am glad you tried to get home on time. We do need to figure out how to deal with Sheila when she's not allowing you to do what you need to do."
Client:	"She does that sometimes, and I don't know what to do."
Therapist:	Good, Lou. That was great! Good job! You stopped. You thought about your options. You chose a good one and then acted. That was excellent. And do you see how the outcome was different?
Client:	Yeah. I'm not sure my Mom would always be that understanding, though.
Therapist:	Like I said, you might be surprised. At the least, it seems worth finding out, doesn't it?
Client:	Yeah.
Therapist:	Why don't we take a look at that situation with your teacher that you mentioned and role-play that one the same way?
Client:	Okay.

Critique of the Anger Control/Problem-Solving Skills Training Demonstration Vignette

The following points were made in the critique:

a. Role-playing and role-reversal are used well by this therapist. Role-playing of the problem-solving technique is a much more powerful teaching technique than simply talking about it.

b. Role-reversal could have been used to teach the teen client empathy for the mother's worry about the child.

c. The therapist generated alternative behaviors that could be used by the client in the situation. It will be helpful in future sessions to have the client brainstorm for alternative reactions to situations that would result in less negative consequences.

d. The therapist makes good use of the sports telecasting example of "freezing the action" to keep ideas at a level close to the teen's interest.

e. The problem-solving approach will have to be applied over and over to new situations before it becomes natural for the teen.

Additional points that could be made:

a. The therapist made good use of verbal reinforcement and encouragement to teach and to build rapport with the client.

b. More could have been made of the client's need to be in control of his emotions during the "stop, think, and act" application of problem-solving. This will be a major adjustment for the explosive client.

Comments you would like to make:

_____

_____

_____

_____

Homework: The homework exercise "Alternatives to Destructive Anger" (*Adult Psychotherapy Homework Planner*, 2nd ed., by Jongsma) is an exercise that highlights constructive alternatives to aggressive anger, such as using assertiveness, calming, problem-solving, and positive self-talk. The assignment "Anger Journal" increases awareness of the prevalence of anger as well as focusing on constructive alternatives. Finally, the exercise "Plan Before Acting" teaches awareness of the negative consequences of impulsive behavior and the advantages of using the problem-solving approach (see www.wiley.com/go/DBehwb).

Skills Training Approaches Review

1. What are common emphases of anger control training approaches to disruptive behavior?

Skills Training Approaches Review Test Question

1. Which of the following is a common catchphrase used to summarily describe the skill set taught to manage anger?

    A. Stop and count to ten

    B. Stop, drop, and roll

    C. Stop, look, and listen

    D. Stop, think, and act

Chapter References

Jongsma, A. E. (2006). *Adult psychotherapy homework planner* (2nd ed.). Hoboken, NJ: Wiley.

Jongsma, A. E., Peterson, L. M., & McInnis, W. P. (2006). *Adolescent therapy homework planner* (2nd ed.). Hoboken, NJ: Wiley.

6

What Are Common Considerations for Relapse Prevention?

Whether treated pharmacologically, psychologically, or both, disruptive behavior, such as that seen in ODD/CD, can relapse. Let's take a look at some common considerations in relapse prevention interventions and how they can be incorporated into your treatment plan.

1. Provide a rationale for relapse prevention that discusses the risk and introduces strategies for preventing it.

   ➤ One of the first steps in relapse prevention interventions is to provide a *rationale* for them. This typically involves a discussion of the risk for relapse and how using the relapse prevention approach we will outline can lower that risk.

2. Discuss with the client the distinction between a lapse and relapse, associating a lapse with a temporary setback and relapse with a return to a sustained pattern of depressive thinking, feeling, interpersonal withdrawal and/or avoidance.

   ➤ Another initial step in this relapse prevention approach is to distinguish between a lapse and relapse. A lapse is presented as a temporary setback that may involve, for example, a behavioral infraction on the child's part, a slip back into an old maladaptive parenting habit, or an initial return of any disruptive behavior.

   ➤ Relapse, on the other hand, is described as a return to a more sustained pattern of disruptive behavior characteristic of ODD/CD.

   ➤ The rationale for this distinction is that a lapse does not need to develop into a relapse if it can be caught and managed.

3. Identify and rehearse managing "high-risk" situations for a lapse.

   ➤ High-risk situations that might make the client vulnerable to a lapse are identified. This discussion may be informed by past difficult experiences or anticipated new ones. Some examples include:

     ➤ When parents are busy, stressed at work, or have unusually high demands on them

➤ When the parent and child have a conflict that is not immediately resolved

➤ When peer pressure is placed on the child to behave disruptively

➤ For the high-risk situations identified, the therapist leads the client in a rehearsal of using skills learned in therapy to manage them, including the skills of developing a tolerance for the lapse while working on how to begin problem-solving them.

4. Instruct the client to routinely use strategies learned in therapy, building them into his/her life as much as possible.

➤ In addition to using skills learned in therapy to manage high-risk situations, parents and children are also encouraged to use strategies learned in therapy during their day-to-day life. Examples include encouraging the consistent use of parent training, problem-solving, assertive communication, anger management, and conflict resolution techniques.

5. Develop a coping card on which coping strategies and other important information can be kept.

➤ Sometimes clients benefit from having a coping card or some other reminder of important strategies and information regarding relapse prevention.

6. Schedule periodic maintenance or "booster" sessions to help the client maintain therapeutic gains and problem-solve challenges.

➤ Periodic booster sessions of therapy can help reinforce positive changes, problem-solve challenges, and facilitate continued improvement, so clients are invited to periodically revisit therapy for these purposes.

Common Considerations in Relapse Prevention

1. Explain the rationale of relapse prevention interventions
2. Distinguish between lapse and relapse
3. Identify and rehearse managing "high-risk" situations for a lapse
4. Encourage routine use of skills learned in therapy
5. Consider developing a coping card
6. Schedule periodic "booster" therapy sessions

Table 6.1 contains examples of how common considerations in relapse prevention could be incorporated into a psychotherapy treatment plan.

Table 6.1   Integrating Relapse Prevention Objective and Interventions into the Treatment Plan

Objective	Interventions
1. Learn and implement strategies to prevent relapse of disruptive behavior.	1. Provide a rationale for relapse prevention that discusses the risk and introduces strategies for preventing it. 2. Discuss with the parent/child the distinction between a lapse and relapse, associating a lapse with a temporary setback and relapse with a return to a sustained pattern of thinking, feeling, and behaving that is characteristic of ODD/CD. 3. Identify and rehearse with the parent/child the management of future situations or circumstances in which lapses could occur. 4. Instruct the parent/child to routinely use strategies learned in therapy (e.g., parent training techniques, problem-solving, anger management), building them into his/her life as much as possible. 5. Develop a coping card on which coping strategies and other important information can be kept (e.g., steps in problem-solving, positive coping statements, reminders that were helpful to the client during therapy). 6. Schedule periodic maintenance or "booster" sessions to help the parent/child maintain therapeutic gains and problem-solve challenges.

Chapter Review

1. What are the common considerations in relapse prevention?

Chapter Review Test Questions

1. The parents of a child and their therapist identify future situations the parents feel could potentially set them back should they occur. They plan to review these encounters and develop a plan for managing them effectively. Which consideration in relapse prevention is being used in this example?

   A. Developing a coping card
   B. Distinguishing between lapse and relapse
   C. Encouraging routine use of skills learned in therapy
   D. Identifying high-risk situations for a lapse

Closing Remarks and Resources

As we note on the DVD, it is important to be aware that the research support for any particular EST supports the identified treatment as it was delivered in the empirical studies. The use of only selected objectives or interventions from ESTs may not be empirically supported.

If you want to incorporate an EST into your treatment plan, it should reflect the major objectives and interventions of the approach. Note that in addition to their primary objectives and interventions, many ESTs have options within them that may or may not be used depending on the client's need (e.g., skills training). Most treatment manuals, books, and other training programs identify the primary objectives and interventions used in the EST.

An existing resource for integrating research-supported treatments into treatment planning is the Practice*Planners*® Series[1] of treatment planners. The series contains several books that have integrated goals, objectives, and interventions consistent with those of identified ESTs into treatment plans for several applicable problems and disorders:

- ➤ *The Severe and Persistent Mental Illness Treatment Planner* (Berghuis, Jongsma, & Bruce)
- ➤ *The Family Therapy Treatment Planner* (Dattilio, Jongsma, & Davis)
- ➤ *The Complete Adult Psychotherapy Treatment Planner* (Jongsma, Peterson, & Bruce)
- ➤ *The Adolescent Psychotherapy Treatment Planner* (Jongsma, Peterson, McInnis, & Bruce)
- ➤ *The Child Psychotherapy Treatment Planner* (Jongsma, Peterson, McInnis, & Bruce)
- ➤ *The Veterans and Active Duty Military Psychotherapy Treatment Planner* (Moore & Jongsma)

---

[1]These books are updated frequently; please check with the publisher for the latest editions and for further information about the Practice*Planners*® series.

➤ *The Addiction Treatment Planner* (Perkinson, Jongsma, & Bruce)
➤ *The Couples Psychotherapy Treatment Planner* (O'Leary, Heyman, & Jongsma)
➤ *The Older Adult Psychotherapy Treatment Planner* (Frazer, Hinrichsen, & Jongsma).

Finally, it is important to remember that the purpose of this series is to demonstrate the process of evidence-based psychotherapy treatment planning for common mental health problems. It is designed to be informational in nature, and does not intend to be a substitute for clinical training in the interventions discussed and demonstrated. In accordance with ethical guidelines, therapists should have competency in the services they deliver.

A Sample Evidence-Based Treatment Plan for Disruptive Behavior

Primary Problem: Oppositional Defiant Behavior

Behavioral Definitions

1. Has a history of explosive, aggressive outbursts
2. Often argues with authority figures over requests or rules
3. Blames others rather than accept responsibility for own problems
4. Displays angry overreaction to perceived disapproval, rejection, or criticism
5. Has a persistent pattern of challenging, resenting, or disrespecting authority figures
6. Uses verbally abusive language
7. Evidences significant impairment in social and academic functioning

Diagnosis: Oppositional Defiant Disorder (313.81)

Long-Term Goals

1. Comply consistently with rules and expectations in the home and school
2. Stop blaming others for problems and accept responsibility for own feelings, thoughts, and behaviors
3. Express anger in a controlled, respectful manner on a consistent basis
4. Parents learn and implement effective child behavioral management skills
5. Reach a level of reduced tension, increased satisfaction, and improved communication with family

Objectives	Interventions
1. Identify major concerns regarding the child's misbehavior and the associated parenting approaches that have been tried.	1. Conduct a clinical interview focused on specifying the nature, severity, and history of the child's misbehavior. 2. Assess how the parents have attempted to respond to the child's misbehavior and what the triggers and reinforcements there may be contributing to the behavior.
2. Describe any conflicts that result from the different approaches to parenting that each partner has.	1. Assess the parent's consistency in their approach to the child and whether they have experienced conflicts between themselves over how to react to the child.

(continued)

Objectives	Interventions
3. Parents and child cooperate with psychological assessment to further delineate the nature of the presenting problem.	1. Administer psychological instruments designed to objectively assess parent-child relational conflict (e.g., the Parent-Child Relationship Inventory [PCRI]); give the clients feedback regarding the results of the assessment; readminister as need to assess outcome. 2. Conduct or arrange for psychological testing to help assess whether a comorbid condition (e.g., depression, Attention Deficit/Hyperactivity Disorder [ADHD]) is contributing to disruptive behavior problems; follow up accordingly with client and parents regarding treatment options; readminister as needed to assess outcome.
4. Cooperate with an evaluation for possible treatment with psychotropic medications to assist in anger and behavioral control and take medications consistently, if prescribed.	1. Assess the client for the need for psychotropic medication to assist in control of anger and other misbehaviors; refer him/her to a physician for an evaluation for prescription medication; monitor prescription compliance, effectiveness, and side effects; provide feedback to the prescribing physician.
5. Verbalize alternative ways to think about and manage anger and misbehavior.	1. Assist the client in conceptualizing his or her disruptive behavior as involving different components (cognitive, physiological, affective, and behavioral) that go through predictable phases that can be managed (e.g., demanding expectations not being met, leading to increased arousal and anger, leading to acting out). 2. Assist the client in identifying the positive consequences of managing anger and misbehavior (e.g., respect from others and self, cooperation from others, improved physical health, etc.); ask the client to agree to learn new ways to conceptualize and manage anger and misbehavior.
6. Parents verbalize an understanding of Parent Management Training, its rationale, and general methods.	1. Describe the Parent Management Training approach to teach the parents how parent and child behavioral interactions can encourage or discourage positive or negative behavior and that changing key elements of those interactions (e.g., prompting and reinforcing positive behaviors) can be used to promote positive change. 2. Ask the parents to read material consistent with a parent training approach to managing disruptive behavior (e.g., *Parenting Through Change* by Forgatch, *Living with Children* by Patterson).
7. Parents implement Parent Management Training skills to identify and reinforce the child's desirable behavior.	1. Teach the parents how to specifically define and identify problem behaviors, identify their own reactions to the behavior, determine whether the reaction encourages or discourages the behavior, and generate alternatives to the problem behavior.

Objectives	Interventions
	2. Assign the parents to implement key parenting practices consistently, including establishing realistic, age-appropriate rules for acceptable and unacceptable behavior; prompting of positive behavior in the environment; use of positive reinforcement to encourage behavior (e.g., praise and clearly established rewards); and use of calm clear direct instruction, time out, and other loss-of-privilege practices for sustained problem behavior.
	3. Assign the parents home exercises in which they implement and record results of implementation exercises (or assign "Clear Rules, Positive Reinforcement, Appropriate Consequences" in the *Brief Adolescent Therapy Homework Planner*, 2nd ed., by Jongsma, Peterson, & McInnis); review in session, providing corrective feedback toward improved, appropriate, and consistent use of skills.
8. Implement Anger Control Training techniques to manage and control anger.	1. Use modeling, role-playing, and behavioral rehearsal to teach the client anger control techniques that include stop, think, and act as well as problem-solving skills; role-play the application of the skills to multiple situations in the client's life.
	2. Assign the client to implement the anger control techniques in his/her daily living; review these incidents; reinforce and provide corrective feedback toward the goal of sustained effective use.
9. Learn and implement strategies to prevent relapse of disruptive behavior.	1. Provide a rationale for relapse prevention that discusses the risk and introduces strategies for preventing it.
	2. Discuss with the parent/child the distinction between a lapse and relapse, associating a lapse with a temporary setback and relapse with a return to a sustained pattern of thinking, feeling, and behaving that is characteristic of ODD/CD.
	3. Identify and rehearse with the parent/child the management of future situations or circumstances in which lapses could occur.
	4. Instruct the parent/child to routinely use strategies learned in therapy (e.g., parent training techniques, problem-solving, anger management), building them into his/her life as much as possible.
	5. Develop a coping card on which coping strategies and other important information can be kept (e.g., steps in problem-solving, positive coping statements, reminders that were helpful to the client during therapy).
	6. Schedule periodic maintenance or "booster" sessions to help the parent/child maintain therapeutic gains and problem-solve challenges.

Chapter Review Test Questions and Answers Explained

Chapter 1: What Are the Disruptive Behavior Disorders?

1. To meet diagnostic criteria such as those in the DSM, what is the minimum length of time that the behavioral characteristics of oppositional defiant disorder (ODD) should be seen in the child?

   A. One month
   B. One year
   C. Six months
   D. Three months
      A. *Incorrect*: The behavioral characteristics of ODD need to be seen longer than one month to meet diagnostic criteria for the disorder.
      B. *Incorrect*: To meet diagnostic criteria for ODD, the behavioral characteristics of it need only be seen for six months.
      C. *Correct*: The behavioral characteristics of ODD need to be seen for at least six months to meet diagnostic criteria for the disorder.
      D. *Incorrect*: The behavioral characteristics of ODD need to be seen longer than three months to meet diagnostic criteria for the disorder.

2. Which of the following is a potentially severe disruptive child/adolescent behavior disorder in which there is often serious violation of the rights of others?

   A. Attention deficit disorder (ADD)
   B. Conduct disorder (CD)
   C. Oppositional defiant disorder (ODD)
   D. Separation anxiety disorder (SAD)
      A. *Incorrect*: Although often disruptive when accompanied by hyperactivity, ADD is not associated with serious violations of the rights of others.

B. *Correct*: The behavior characteristic of CD is associated with serious violations of the rights of others.

C. *Incorrect*: Although often disruptive, ODD is characterized more by noncompliance than with serious violations of the rights of others.

D. *Incorrect*: Although it can be disruptive, SAD is characterized more by fear and avoidance than by serious violations of the rights of others.

Chapter 2: What Are the Six Steps in Building a Treatment Plan?

1. Although all are disruptive, children with ODD may be disruptive in different ways. For example, some may argue and defy adults predominately, while others may deliberately annoy and blame peers. In which step of treatment planning would you record the particular expressions of ODD for your client?

A. Creating short-term objectives
B. Describing the problem's manifestations
C. Identifying the primary problem
D. Selecting treatment interventions

A. *Incorrect*: Arguing, defying, annoying, and the like are expressions or symptom manifestations of ODD, not objectives for the client to achieve.

B. *Correct*: Features, also referred to as expressions or manifestations, of a problem for the particular client are described in Step 2 of treatment planning: describing the problem's manifestations.

C. *Incorrect*: Arguing, defying, annoying, and the like are expressions or symptom manifestations of the primary problem of ODD.

D. *Incorrect*: Arguing, defying, annoying, and the like are expressions or symptom manifestations of ODD, not a therapist's action designed to help the client achieve his or her objective(s).

2. The statement, "Learn Parent Management techniques to identify and reinforce the child's desirable behavior," is an example of which of the following steps in a treatment plan?

A. A primary problem
B. A short-term objective
C. A symptom manifestation
D. A treatment intervention

A. *Incorrect*: The primary problem (Step 1 in Treatment Planning) is the summary description, usually in diagnostic terms, of the client's primary problem.

B. *Correct*: This is a short-term objective (Step 5 in Treatment Planning). It describes the desired actions of the client in the treatment plan.

    C. *Incorrect*: Symptom manifestations (Step 2 in Treatment Planning) describe the client's particular expression (i.e., manifestations or symptoms) of a problem.

    D. *Incorrect*: A treatment intervention (Step 6 in Treatment Planning) describes the therapist's actions designed to help the client achieve therapeutic objectives.

Chapter 3: What Is the Brief History of the Empirically Supported Treatments Movement?

1. Which statement best describes the process used to identify ESTs?

    A. Consumers of mental health services nominated therapies.

    B. Experts came to a consensus based on their experiences with the treatments.

    C. Researchers submitted their works.

    D. Task groups reviewed the literature using clearly defined selection criteria for ESTs.

        A. *Incorrect*: Mental health professionals selected ESTs.

        B. *Incorrect*: Expert consensus was not the method used to identify ESTs.

        C. *Incorrect*: Empirical works in the existing literature were reviewed to identify ESTs.

        D. *Correct*: Review groups consisting of mental health professionals selected ESTs based on predetermined criteria such as *well-established* and *probably efficacious*.

2. Based on the differences in their criteria, in which of the following ways are well-established treatments different than those classified as probably efficacious?

    A. Only probably efficacious treatments allowed the use of a single case design experiment.

    B. Only well-established treatments allowed studies comparing the treatment to a psychological placebo.

    C. Only well-established treatments required demonstration by at least two different, independent investigators or investigating teams.

    D. Only well-established treatments allowed studies comparing the treatment to a pill placebo.

        A. *Incorrect*: Both sets of criteria allowed use of single subject designs. Well-established treatments required a larger series than did probably efficacious treatments (see II under Well-Established and III under Probably Efficacious).

        B. *Incorrect*: Studies using comparison to psychological placebos were acceptable in both sets of criteria (see IA under Well-Established and II under Probably Efficacious).

C. *Correct*: One of the primary differences between treatments classified as well-established and those classified as probably efficacious is that well-established therapies have had their efficacy demonstrated by at least two different, independent investigators (see V under Well-Established).

D. *Incorrect*: Studies using comparison to pill placebos were acceptable in both sets of criteria (see IA under Well-Established and II under Probably Efficacious).

Chapter 4: What Are the Identified Empirically Supported Treatments for the Disruptive Behavior Disorders?

1. Empirically supported treatments for oppositional and defiant behavior in younger children (age 8 or younger) typically emphasize which of the following?

   A. Teaching the child anger management skills
   B. Teaching the child problem-solving skills
   C. Training parents in child management skills
   D. Training peers who then help the child

      A. *Incorrect*: This intervention is typical when working with older children and adolescents.

      B. *Incorrect*: This intervention is typical when working with older children and adolescents.

      C. *Correct*: This intervention is typical when working with younger children.

      D. *Incorrect*: This intervention is used sometimes when working with older children and adolescents.

2. Which of the following therapeutic approaches identified by APA's Division 53 meets the criteria for a well-established EST?

   A. Anger control training
   B. Assertiveness training
   C. Problem-solving skills training
   D. Parent management training

      A. *Incorrect*: Although having demonstrated efficacy for the treatment of disruptive behavior, this intervention has not met the criteria for a well-established treatment used by APA's Division 12 and requiring independent replication.

      B. *Incorrect*: Although having demonstrated efficacy for the treatment of disruptive behavior, this intervention has not met the criteria for a well-established treatment used by APA's Division 12 and requiring independent replication.

C. *Incorrect*: Although having demonstrated efficacy for the treatment of disruptive behavior, this intervention has not met the criteria for a well-established treatment used by APA's Division 12 and requiring independent replication.

D. *Correct*: Parent management is the only treatment for disruptive behavior that has demonstrated efficacy, meeting the criteria for a well-established treatment used by APA's Division 12 and requiring independent replication.

Chapter 5: How Do You Integrate ESTs into Treatment Planning?

Assessment/Psychoeducation

1. At what point in therapy is psychoeducation conducted?

   A. At the end of therapy
   B. During the assessment phase
   C. During the initial treatment session
   D. Throughout therapy

      A. *Incorrect*: Although there may be some psychoeducation done at this phase of therapy, psychoeducation is conducted throughout therapy.
      B. *Incorrect*: Although there is commonly some psychoeducation done at assessment, psychoeducation is conducted throughout therapy.
      C. *Incorrect*: Although it is common for psychoeducation to be done early in therapy, it continues throughout.
      D. *Correct*: Psychoeducation permeates all phases of therapy.

Parent Management Training

1. Which of the following practices is most consistent with Parent Management Training (PMT)?

   A. Identifying and punishing undesirable behavior
   B. Identifying and rewarding desirable behavior
   C. Teaching disruptive children anger management skills
   D. Teaching disruptive children problem-solving skills

      A. *Incorrect*: Emphasis in PMT is on reinforcing prosocial behavior. Response cost intervention (e.g., removing a privilege) may be used for persistent misbehavior. Punishment is not.
      B. *Correct*: The emphasis in PMT is positively reinforcing desired child behavior.

   C. *Incorrect*: This approach better characterizes skill-building approaches
      to disruptive behavior in older children and adolescents.
   D. *Incorrect*: This approach better characterizes skill-building approaches
      to disruptive behavior in older children and adolescents.

Skills Training Approaches

1. Which of the following is a common catchphrase used to summarily describe
   the skill set taught to manage anger?

   A. Stop and count to ten
   B. Stop, drop, and roll
   C. Stop, look, and listen
   D. Stop, think, and act
      A. *Incorrect*: This may be helpful in stopping oneself from further escalat-
         ing an angry reaction, but it's not the catchphrase for the essence of the
         anger management approach.
      B. *Incorrect*: This is what you do if your clothes are on fire.
      C. *Incorrect*: This is what you're supposed to do before crossing a street.
      D. *Correct*: Although the phrase doesn't capture all that's involved in man-
         aging anger, it's commonly used to summarize the key features of the
         approach—and sometimes helps clients remember them.

Chapter 6: What Are Common Considerations for Relapse Prevention?

1. The parents of a child and their therapist identify future situations the parents
   feel could potentially set them back should they occur. They plan to review
   these encounters and develop a plan for managing them effectively. Which consideration in relapse prevention is being used in this example?

   A. Developing a coping card
   B. Distinguishing between lapse and relapse
   C. Encouraging routine use of skills learned in therapy
   D. Identifying high-risk situations for a lapse
      A. *Incorrect*: This is a technique used by some clients to help them remem-
         ber key therapeutic points and strategies outside of therapy.
      B. *Incorrect*: This is a psychoeducational intervention designed in part to
         help prevent misinterpretation of potentially manageable "setbacks" as
         an unmanageable relapse.
      C. *Incorrect*: This intervention is designed to transport skill use into every-
         day applications, not just ones that represent a higher risk for relapse.
      D. *Correct*: The vignette describes identifying high-risk situations. James and
         his therapist will then review and develop a plan for managing them.

STUDY PACKAGE
CONTINUING EDUCATION
CREDIT INFORMATION

Evidence-Based Treatment Planning for Disruptive Child & Adolescent Behavior

Our goal is to provide you with current, accurate and practical information from the most experienced and knowledgeable speakers and authors.

Listed below are the continuing education credit(s) currently available for this self-study package. *Please note: Your state licensing board dictates whether self study is an acceptable form of continuing education. Please refer to your state rules and regulations.*

COUNSELORS: PESI, LLC is recognized by the National Board for Certified Counselors to offer continuing education for National Certified Counselors. Provider #: 5896. We adhere to NBCC Continuing Education Guidelines. This self-study package qualifies for **1.0** contact hours.

SOCIAL WORKERS: PESI, LLC, 1030, is approved as a provider for continuing education by the Association of Social Work Boards, 400 South Ridge Parkway, Suite B, Culpeper, VA 22701. www.aswb. org. Social workers should contact their regulatory board to determine course approval. Course Level: All Levels. Social Workers will receive **1.0** (Clinical) continuing education clock hours for completing this self-study package.

PSYCHOLOGISTS: PESI, LLC is approved by the American Psychological Association to sponsor continuing education for psychologists. PESI, LLC maintains responsibility for these materials and their content. PESI is offering these self- study materials for **1.0** hours of continuing education credit.

ADDICTION COUNSELORS: PESI, LLC is a Provider approved by NAADAC Approved Education Provider Program. Provider #: 366. This self-study package qualifies for **1.0** contact hours.

Procedures:

1. Review the material and read the book.

2. If seeking credit, complete the posttest/evaluation form:

    -Complete posttest/evaluation in entirety; including your email address to receive your certificate much faster versus by mail.

    -Upon completion, mail to the address listed on the form along with the CE fee stated on the test. Tests will not be processed without the CE fee included.

    -Completed posttests must be received 6 months from the date printed on the packing slip.

Your completed posttest/evaluation will be graded. If you receive a passing score (70% and above), you will be emailed/faxed/mailed a certificate of successful completion with earned continuing education credits. (Please write your email address on the posttest/evaluation form for fastest response) If you do not pass the posttest, you will be sent a letter indicating areas of deficiency, and another posttest to complete. The posttest must be resubmitted and receive a passing grade before credit can be awarded. We will allow you to re-take as many times as necessary to receive a certificate.

If you have any questions, please feel free to contact our customer service department at 1.800.844.8260.

PESI LLC
PO BOX 1000
Eau Claire, WI 54702-1000

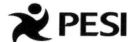 **PESI**

Evidence-Based Treatment Planning for Disruptive
Child & Adolescent Behavior

PO BOX 1000
Eau Claire, WI 54702
800-844-8260

Any persons interested in receiving credit may photocopy this form, complete and return with a payment of $15.00 per person CE fee. A certificate of successful completion will be sent to you. To receive your certificate sooner than two weeks, rush processing is available for a fee of $10. Please attach check or include credit card information below.

Mail to: PESI, PO Box 1000, Eau Claire, WI 54702 or fax to PESI (800) 554-9775 (both sides)

CE Fee: $15: (Rush processing fee: $10)   **Total to be charged** _____

Credit Card #: _____   **Exp Date:** _____ **V-Code*:** _____
(*MC/VISA/Discover: last 3-digit # on signature panel on back of card.) (*American Express: 4-digit # above account # on face of card.)

	LAST	FIRST	M.I.

Name (please print): _____   _____ _____

Address: _____ Daytime Phone: _____

City: _____ State: _____ Zip Code: _____

Signature: _____ Email: _____

Date Completed: _____ Actual time (# of hours) taken to complete this offering: _____hours

Program Objectives After completing this publication, I have been able to achieve these objectives:

1. Explain the process and criteria for diagnosing the disruptive behavior disorders.   1. Yes   No

2. List the six steps in building a clear psychotherapy treatment plan.   2. Yes   No

3. Examine how empirically supported treatments for disruptive behavior disorders have been identified.   3. Yes   No

4. Examine the objectives and treatment interventions consistent with those of identified empirically supported treatments for disruptive behavior disorders.   4. Yes   No

5. Explain how to construct a psychotherapy treatment plan and inform it with objectives and treatment interventions consistent with those identified empirically supported treatments for disruptive behavior disorders.   5. Yes   No

6. Identify common considerations in the prevention of relapse of disruptive behavior disorders.   6. Yes   No

PESI LLC
PO BOX 1000
Eau Claire, WI 54702-1000

ZNT043340   CE Release Date: 2/11/2011

Participant Profile:
1. Job Title: _____ Employment setting: _____

1. According to psychiatric diagnostic classification systems, which of the following child/adolescent disorders is characterized by a serious pattern of repetitive and persistently defiant behaviors in which the basic rights of others or major age-appropriate societal norms or rules are violated?
A. Attention deficit disorder
B. Conduct disorder
C. Oppositional defiant disorder
D. Separation anxiety disorder

2. Jonathan is an 8-year-old boy who often refuses to comply and argues with adults' requests. With peers, he is often witnessed deliberately annoying them, blaming them for his mistakes, and feeling angry and resentful. This pattern of behavior has been witnessed over the last 10 months by his teachers, who report that Jonathan is not adapting well to school. Which of the following diagnoses best fits this pattern of behavior?
A. Attention deficit disorder with hyperactivity
B. Conduct disorder
C. Oppositional defiant disorder
D. Separation anxiety disorder

3. In reference to question 2, Jonathan's refusal to comply, his arguments with adults, and his blaming of others represent which of the following features of a psychotherapy treatment plan?
A. Behavioral definitions
B. Primary problems
C. Short-term objective
D. Therapeutic interventions

4. As discussed in this program, which of the following requirements was unique to APA Division 12's criteria for a well-established treatment, differentiating it from lesser levels of evidence such as probably efficacious?
A. Independent replication of efficacy studies was required.
B. Use of pill placebos in efficacy studies was required.
C. Use of psychological placebos in efficacy studies was required.
D. Use of random assignment in efficacy studies was required.

5. According to the review of the Society of Clinical Child and Adolescent Psychology (APA Division 53) discussed in this program, which of the following treatment approaches for disruptive behavior meets the criteria for a well-established treatment?
A. Anger control training
B. Group assertiveness training
C. Behavioral parent training
D. Problem-solving skills training

6. According to this program, which of the following research-supported treatments are most appropriate for disruptive behavior in young children (8 years old and younger)?
A. Anger control training and group assertiveness training
B. Anger control training and problem-solving skills training
C. Group assertiveness training and problem-solving skills training
D. Parent-child interaction training and parent management training

7. Lou is a 15-year-old boy with oppositional behavior often related to frustration he expresses about his parents' rules. Lou's therapist is teaching him how to stop and consider various options for responding when frustrated. They weigh the pros and cons of each option and select the option they believe will be most adaptive. This intervention characterizes a primary feature of which research-supported treatment for disruptive behavior?
A. Group assertiveness training
B. Multisystemic therapy
C. Parent management training
D. Problem-solving skills training

8. A therapist helps the parents of a disruptive child implement key parenting practices consistently, including establishing realistic age-appropriate rules for acceptable and unacceptable behavior, prompting of positive behavior in the environment, and use of positive reinforcement to encourage acceptable behavior. These practices are consistent with which research-supported treatment for disruptive behavior?
A. Anger control training
B. Multisystemic therapy
C. Parent management training
D. Problem-solving skills training

9. According to this program, an intervention commonly used in relapse prevention is to help the client incorporate the skills learned through therapy into his or her everyday life.
A. TRUE
B. FALSE

10. Which of the following best describes the approach to creating an evidence-based treatment plan for disruptive behavior disorders that is recommended in this program?
A. The therapist conducts group assertiveness skills training.
B. The therapist conducts parent-child interaction therapy.
C. The therapist incorporates into therapy the objectives and interventions consistent with research-supported treatments for disruptive behavior disorders.
D. The therapist incorporates into therapy the use of an objective measure of disruptive behavior to track treatment progress.

PESI LLC PO BOX 1000 Eau Claire, WI 54702-1000